BRADY

Prehospital Documentation

AF704187

BRADY

Prehospital Documentation

A Systematic Approach

Armando S. Bevelacqua

Firefighter/Paramedic
Educator/Consultant

BRADY
A Prentice Hall Division
Englewood Cliffs, NJ 07632

Library of Congress Cataloging–in–Publication Data

Bevelacqua, Armando S.,
Prehospital documentation : a systematic approach / Armando S. Bevelacqua.
p. cm.
ISBN 0–89303–948–9
1. Communication in emergency medicine. 2. Medical writing.
I. Title.
RC86.3.B48 1992
616.02′5—dc20 91–39630
CIP

Editorial/production supervision
and interior design: *Julie Boddorf*
Cover design: *Wanda Lubelska*
Prepress buyer: *Ilene Levy*
Manufacturing buyer: *Ed O'Dougherty*
Acquisitions editor: *Natalie Anderson*
Editorial assistant: *Louise Fullam*

Printed in the United States of America

ISBN 0-89303-948-9

Prentice-Hall International (UK) Limited, *London*
Prentice-Hall of Australia Pty. Limited, *Sydney*
Prentice-Hall Canada Inc., *Toronto*
Prentice-Hall Hispanoamericana, S.A., *Mexico*
Prentice-Hall of India Private Limited, *New Delhi*
Prentice-Hall of Japan, Inc., *Tokyo*
Simon & Schuster Asia Pte. Ltd., *Singapore*
Editora Prentice-Hall do Brasil, Ltda., *Rio de Janeiro*

To
Brianne and Nicholas

This manual belongs to ______________________________

Home Address ______________________________

Department/Address ______________________________

Shift/Station ______________________________

Important Emergency Telephone Numbers:

Dispatch Communications : ______________________________

E.D. ______________ : ______________________________

E.D. ______________ : ______________________________

E.D. ______________ : ______________________________

E.D. ______________ : ______________________________

E.D. ______________ : ______________________________

E.D. ______________ : ______________________________

Station # ______________ : ______________________________

Station # ______________ : ______________________________

Station # ______________ : ______________________________

Station # ______________ : ______________________________

Station # ______________ : ______________________________

Station # ______________ : ______________________________

Station # ______________ : ______________________________

______________ : ______________________________

______________ : ______________________________

______________ : ______________________________

______________ : ______________________________

______________ : ______________________________

______________ : ______________________________

Contents

Preface

Since the beginning of EMS, the EMT/paramedic has been striving for a place in the professional spotlight. Don't look now, but the light is on and is shining very brightly! EMT/paramedics are now licensed/certified in some states. With this "licensing/certification" comes a definable responsibility: We are medically and legally accountable for our actions. We are the people who start the IVs or intubate the patient, decide how, when, and where the patient is to be transported, and we are the ones who load the patient into the transporting vehicle. Because we are the first on the scene, our actions have a direct impact on the outcome, the well-being, if not the very lives of our patients.

The emergency medical field is no longer under the Good Samaritan mantle. We are now in the professional arena, and as such, we must communicate on a professional level. It is true that our actions have been observed by both our training instructors and medical director; however, once we are in the field, we are the first ones "calling the shots," not the training instructor, not the medical director. If we make a mistake, it is our mistake, not the physician's. The actions performed and the decisions made are the EMT/paramedic's responsibility and no one else.

Do not assume that because your system has protocols, the system will protect you. You are wrong. Your judgment must be derived from sound medical fact (your training and in-service education) and what has been observed (your protocols and the experience to apply them). Standards and procedures were developed over many years, forming a common body of knowledge, a foundation. These gradually became more involved until they emerged as concepts that are now acknowledged as mandatory practice. If there is a deviation from this absolute routine, a standard has been breached; the EMS provider has become negligent, which could, at a later date be considered malpractice. Proper documentation—report writing—becomes critical.

When writing a report you are, in effect, describing everything that happened while you were with the patient or patients. The person reading your report should be able to reconstruct the incident without any doubt as to the details of what actually took place. The order in which we report the events are equally important. Sentence structure should not be flowery, but rather, precise, direct, and informative. You are not writing a speech. You are an EMS provider. Get to the point and stick with it. Wordy expressions tend to cloud the facts, putting doubt in the mind of the reader. If there is any uncertainty as to what took place, be assured that your report can be questioned at a later date. A well-written report can ensure the level of credibility of your agency as well as yourself. Remember, a report can be used as testimony in a court of law, and you will be expected to state what happened without any deviation from what was written.

Military and civilian physicians have recognized the expertise of the EMS provider. The knowledge base of EMTs/paramedics is unmatched. Their experience at rapid triage, crisis intervention, and decision making is something that is not learned in books, but rather is developed from repetitive exposure to the types of cases that require fast, invasive, and precise judgment. This is judgment required without the benefit of a lengthy discussion or consultation—and physicians recognize this.

We as prehospital care providers have been trained to observe and to act on what we see, do, or find. We are the first to record and document medical facts as well as other observations. Once we have accumulated this body of critical information, it is passed on to the receiving physician. After a limited interaction with the doctor, further orders are given and performed. All along, a written document is being assembled. This document will follow the patient and become part of the patient's written medical history, both legally and medically. What we saw, did, and found becomes fact—verifiable fact and thus considered evidence. Because it is evidence the report and the persons involved in that report can be subpoenaed into a court of law (and the medical report now becomes legal evidence). Unless all facts related to the incident are properly documented and comprehensively recorded, the result can be a medic's (as well as an agency's) nightmare.

The business world is based on the art of communication, both verbal and written. With the growing use of computers and telecommunications within all the disciplines, the ability to observe, describe, and record the interactions of others now becomes critical to the job of the emergency worker. For many years the name, age, and a brief description of the patient's complaint was all that was required. This has now changed dramatically. Instead, rescue workers are called to present themselves in a court under subpoena, sometimes many years after the incident, to state under oath what was said to the patient, how the patient was found, who might have been in the room or on the scene, and even possibly at what time intervention was started. Because recollection is not that reliable, it is inconceivable that we can pull out of memory what we did four years ago at 1130 hours, November 11. Therefore, records have to be kept, documenting pertinent information relating to each particular incident. It is a document that should not be taken lightly.

What was once thought of the trappings of the business world is now EMS reality. We are required to become proficient communicators of the written word. While system evaluation has been on the desk of all EMS managers, a measuring stick has never been established outlining the specifics of EMS reporting. Quality assurance programs will eventually establish such tools of measurement. It is therefore of immediate concern to raise the quality of documentation, making it within the skill and scope of every prehospital provider. Quality assurance has become a hot buzzword of the business world. It is now considered part of all professional responsibility.

A report should be clear, brief, and complete as well as accurate. It must have the appropriate classifications and should be objectively informative. It is my desire to provide such a guide: an approach that will enable you, the prehospital provider, to do just that.

NOTE: *It is the intent of the authors and publisher that this book be used as part of a formal education program taught by a qualified instructor and supervised by a licensed physician. The care procedures presented here represent accepted practices in the United States. They are not offered as a standard of care. Emergency care is to be performed* **only** *under the authority and guidance of a licensed physician. It is the reader's responsibility to know and follow local care protocols as provided by medical advisors directing the system to which he or she belongs. Also, it is the reader's responsibility to stay informed of emergency care procedure changes.*

ACKNOWLEDGMENTS

I would like to take this opportunity to say thanks to the countless students I have instructed over the years. Their input and astute questioning have contributed much not only to this book but to the EMS field in total.

Many people have generously shared their ideas and comments in reviewing this book. Their experience, time, and critique helped determine the final format of this publication. At the top of the list is a group of people to whom I am especially indebted: Chief Ed Hesse, Chief Dave Freeman, and Engineer/Paramedic John Lasseter. We worked together at the same time, in the same office, and shared many invaluable experiences. Our endless hours of discussions and "think tank team" approach to many problems are reflected herein.

Since the inception of my idea on report writing, Natalie Anderson and Louise Fullam, both of the Brady Company, have played an instrumental role in the logistics of idea conception. Their encouragement is most appreciated. They have become supportive with their comments, and their ready interchange of ideas brought to light different avenues and possible approaches.

When publishing a text, obstacles sometimes influence the way textbooks are written. Thanks to the editorial and production assistance of Julie Boddorf, my intent of the manuscript was maintained. A warm thank you to all the unmentioned personnel at Brady that were involved with this production.

I am grateful to Dave Bruton for his suggestions and input on the generic report. His computer background was invaluable to this project, not to mention his creativity. Thanks, Dave!

Last but not least, I thank my wife Grace for putting up with an enormous amount of paperwork, which all but obliterated our dining room table.

To everyone, including my parents for the interest in knowledge, creativity, and books which they instilled in me as a child, I give thanks.

ABOUT THE AUTHOR

Armando S. Bevelacqua has been involved with prehospital care for the past seventeen years. Within this time he has functioned as a flight medic, supervisor aboard a mobile intensive care unit, and as a technician within an emergency room and cardiac intensive care unit. He has worked for the private-sector ambulance and civil service. For the last eight years he has been involved with quality assurance programs and prehospital care instruction (both EMT and paramedic level). He currently holds a position with Valencia Community College instructing EMTs and is involved with continuing education.

He is codirector and cofounder of Emergency Management Systems, a firm specializing in hazardous materials medical training. His company provides training and consultant services to emergency medical services, fire departments, and hospital agencies.

He currently serves as a firefighter/paramedic with the City of Orlando Fire Department, Orlando, Florida. His assigned duties hold him responsible for the quality assurance program and documentation review, along with primary fire/rescue response, hazardous materials responder (technician level), and high-angle tactical response team.

Introduction

Report writing is a skill, and like any skill, can be mastered through diligent application. Once we are aware of what comprises a "good" report, we are on the way to excellence. There are no hard-and-fast rules pertaining to report writing. There are, however certain elements that will make one report better than another; one type of format is not necessarily better than another. There are so many elements to be considered that it is easy in an emergency situation to overlook several factors that can become stumbling blocks in the future.

Documentation can be in the form of notes, footnotes, or a biography of the incident. Field reports are not conducive to this type of technical writing, but rather, need the same high degree of accuracy that technical reports have.

Most departments use a general preprinted report or a standard form. This general format is highly useful for rapidly recording the events of a medical incident. However, the medical information is sketchy at best and needs additional comments (written description) as to the actual events that took place. Much of the needed information is captured within the general format, but because the written report presents an overwhelming task, the following guidelines will enable you to write a highly technical, accurate, and concise field medical report that will clearly include all the necessary facts.

This reference guide is for easy use in report writing. Some of the categories are repeats of previous areas; however, they are repeated to provide a complete picture within each category eliminating the necessity of cross-reference. In using the reference guide, one of three methods may be employed: the head-to-toe, body systems, or call incident approach.

The head-to-toe section is well used with the other two approaches and can also stand alone. It "looks" at the situation in very much the same way that one would perform a head-to-toe survey, documenting the positive findings along with the negative ones.

In the body systems approach method to report writing, the person determines the body system(s) that are affected for the particular observed response. You turn to the system that is being affected, using the systems section and the head-to-toe section, in conjunction with each other. Under the appropriate system there is a list of items to be observed, checked, reevaluated, and documented.

With the call incident approach, the rescue worker turns to the type of incident into which the call may fall. This category outlines criteria that should be observed, evaluated, and reevaluated. Criteria for possible consideration are also listed. At the end of the call incident is a list of observations/skills performed with the necessary responses that should be observed and most important, documented. For further assistance, a spelling dictionary, anatomical charts, and scoring charts have been included which will aid the rescuer in generating a professional, accurate, and concise field report.

I trust the formats presented here will help organize your thoughts when writing your reports while aiding you in remembering a "list" of objectives that one should always consider when taking care of patients. This book is not a set or finished product, but rather a beginning. It is a manual that will change and develop over time according to our needs. It is a guide, intended to help you write reports like a professional.

Because of the status of emergency work and the climate for quick legal recourse, the need for thoroughness in documentation cannot be overemphasized. It is my intent that such a reference guide will serve this function. However, to do this, meeting the needs of all who use this book, feedback is essential. If something is not mentioned or is not clearly written, please feel free to write to me through the publisher, so that future editions can include and encompass all the information that we can garnish from a mass of individual responses and experiences in the field. It is my hope that through the students and instructors who use this book, we will be able to identify future needs.

A.S.B.

BRADY

Prehospital Documentation

1

Effective Report Writing

Documentation covers a large discipline, encompassing a vast amount of material, making it impractical to consider fully all aspects within the confines of one text. The subject to be fully covered in this book is the written medical report, commonly referred as a *report writing*.

For many years the prehospital world has seen less documentation and justification than any combined business found in the corporate sector. The main reason for this is that money constraints and litigation have only recently entered the prehospital environment. For the first time in emergency medical service (EMS) history, the run report has become the sole shred of evidence for the prehospital provider.

Before I embarked on this project, I only considered the necessity of documenting properly, a need that was not addressed in the prehospital curriculum. I looked for classes in such a discipline and soon found nothing that applied to the EMS field specifically. I felt the need to develop an approach, a system that would be accurate, simple, and complete. To this end I sought to educate myself in every facet. The result is an approach that is time saving, easy to remember, and easy to use, as well as a handy practical reference book for resource material and/or unusual information.

Since the inception of EMS, emergency medical technicians and paramedics have functioned as an extension of the emergency room's trusting hands. However, within today's climate of easy lawsuits and under the critical eye of a plaintiff's attorney retained by a poor and/or injured client, inadequately reported facts of lifesaving procedures can be misconstrued or distorted to portray a negative picture. Never intended to be used in a court of law, facts noted to save time in order to benefit the patient and to acquaint the physician quickly with the patient's condition and the emergency procedures involved now become a tool for an attorney with just enough evidence for wide-open speculation.

In times past the only person reviewing such a report was the originator himself or herself. Times have changed; the number of personnel reading your report on the average might be as few as four: yourself, your immediate supervisor, quality assurance personnel, and the report clerk—each checking for legibility, accuracy, and clarity. However, if the incident goes to court, you have now magnified the number of interested reviewers three- or four-fold, and perhaps more. What is written down is judged good or bad, right or wrong, and what was not stated (whatever the reason) will be considered as never having been performed. The report can be the ultimate double-edged sword.

Documentation also supports justification. In times of money constraints, recessions, and the general economic climate upon which EMS monies are allocated, justification becomes essential to the continuance and furtherance of the service. Like any well-designed reporting system, justification can be provided if designed properly. Justification also involves the legal system, justification of equipment, justification of personnel, quality assurance, and total system analysis, to name a few. For the purposes of this book it will be mentioned only as it pertains to the subject on hand—report writing.

When I first came up with an organized approach to the report-writing technique, I had several lists that did not make sense to anyone but me. I still had trouble remembering all the details one had to include in a written report. I thought if I were to present this to my peers, giving them a workable approach, one that they could relate to, it would have to be simple and the information would have to be easy to find and easy to remember. After writing many reports and spending much time analyzing the problem, teaching aspiring persons to become EMTs and paramedics, and out of much talk with students, peers, and medical professionals, the approach presented here incorporates the basics of EMS: the head-to-toe survey—with some modifications and alterations.

All three approaches utilize the head-to-toe concept in one way or another. In each category and approach I have included other possibilities and considerations. You are not going to use all the information that is presented within each category; however, in each approach I present items that should be considered, and if applicable, documented.

There are four avenues or methods that can be used (or followed):

1. **SOAP** method
2. **CHARTE** method
3. **Body systems approach**
4. **MIV** method

Each method has its own merits.

SOAP Method

No one method is better than another, nor are they the only possible formats that can be used. I know that these four approaches work. If you have developed a format that works for you, keep it, use it, perhaps modify it if necessary. I am presenting these formats primarily for those persons who have a difficult time organizing their thoughts, actions, and findings into words. Secondarily, I present these formats for those people who have a routine way of documenting that is not complete enough to cover the situation in the line of present-day needs for legal documentation. All documentation must be complete as well as accurate.

I personally like the SOAP method, because it is easy to use and seems to be the overall type of reporting that has been successful and has received the most approval from the medical–legal field. It presents the picture you are trying to convey in a simple and logical manner.

S **Subjective.** The history of the patient: both immediate history and the precipitating events, medications, and reactions—basically, what the patient has told you.

O **Objective.** What you as the rescuer have found; this includes the primary and secondary assessment.

A **Assessment** of the incident as a whole. Not a diagnosis but rather a general impression of the condition(s) presented.

P **Plan** of action. Basically, the treatment that was given to your patient.

SOAP gives the reader a format by which all inclusive information is gathered fast and efficiently. If one wants to read the assessment rather than the treatment, he or she does not have to waste time reading a lot of irrelevant information. We discuss SOAP in more detail later.

CHARTE Method

This category of documentation is similar to the SOAP format; however, we have divided the subjective into two parts and the treatment into two areas. The one advantage this format provides is a place to document problems seemingly always present at an EMS scene.

C **Chief Complaint.** What the patient tells you—his or her description of the incident or problem.

H **History.** The patient's immediate history and any precipitating events; medications would be included.

A **Assessment.** The full assessment, primary and secondary.

R **Treatment.** The treatment that was given prior to the arrival of the EMS unit, and scene treatment.

T **Transport.** The treatment that was given enroute to the medical facility and the mode of that transportation.

E **Exceptions.** The problems that were encountered during the incident.

The advantage to the CHARTE format is that it breaks down the incident into logical parts. It distinguishes among assessment, what was found, and the treatment given both on the scene and enroute to the hospital. This is an area that many prehospital providers neglect to include but which is necessary that the physician be aware of.

The disadvantage is that you are not always going to use the total format, leaving blanks that might confuse the reader and bringing up the question: Why was this not completed? Although this method is not well known, it is getting great reviews. In some settings information may be incomplete due to the format's unfamiliarity. However, it does present an organized report, a thorough analysis of all available facts.

Body Systems Approach

This method of documentation is probably the most conclusive of all the methods; however, in its pure form it is difficult to apply in the field. Within this method all systems are evaluated and documented very much like the nursing assessments that are presented in most texts. It is an approach that is time consuming. What I have done is to take this basic approach and incorporate the EMS method of rapid evaluation to satisfy two disciplines: the nursing discipline, in its approach to gaining large and conclusive information, and the EMS prehospital discipline, by gathering a rapid systems assessment.

Where this differs from the nursing system is that it hones in on the system or systems that are directly affected—unlike the total systems approach in nursing, which would include all systems, regardless of the system(s) effected or affected.

More about this later when we combine the formats with the approach that I have developed.

MIV Method

The last format, brief and to the point, is at the other end of the spectrum. It is the least informative and leaves a lot of vital information out. However, despite its incompleteness, it does have a place within the prehospital arena.

M **Mechanism of Injury.** The events that precipitated the incident you were called to.

I **Injury.** The injury itself or the precipitating problems or events (i.e., the head-to-toe survey).

V **Vitals.** Current vitals or a brief description of vital sign changes.

It does not give the amount of information the other formats give, nor does it organize thoughts. However, it does present the incident in a very concise manner, one that can be adapted to the communication that is given via radio. The intent of this type of format is to give the listener a condensed description of the scene and the patient in logical order. The reason is to obtain orders for patient care or notification of patient load to the receiving facility. It works extremely well in mass casualty incidents, allowing the receiving institution to triage patients and prepare for possible treatment priorities.

To provide a feeling for the information needed and the considerations available to you, I would like next to discuss the report categories.

ASSESSMENT: REPORT CATEGORIES

"Where do we start?" The biggest question most EMS providers ask themselves: "What is important, and to what level do I document?" These are some of the questions that I wanted to have answered myself and which led primarily to the writing of this book.

If you take a glance at the assessment area, you might ask yourself: "Do I need all this information all the time?" The answer is no. In some incidents, the information presented will help you document what went on; at other times you might use only a small portion of the ideas on hand. The term *assessment* is not to imply that this is how you assessed your patient; all it is doing is reviewing a list of possibilities that one may use. For example, with a pediatric patient you might have done a toe-to-head survey; however, when writing your report you may document your assessment from the head to the toes.

We have to think of our documentation as a "story." For our story to make sense, we must not leave anything out. Just like a story, a report must have a logical beginning and a logical conclusion. The meat of the matter is in the middle. It has to make sense to both the one writing the report and the one that must read the report—to the one at the scene as well as the one reviewing the scene and the report. The beginning of our story outlines the basic facts that initiated the response of the emergency vehicles: *why* you were sent to this location, *when* the participating event took place, *who* was involved, *where* it happened, and *what* took place prior to EMS arrival. In all of the categories we find that the initial area provides the history of the patient, as well as what precipitated the incident. Basically, all documentation must include why you were called and the needs of the patient. Whichever category we use, these questions must be answered.

The next area necessary to documentation are the baseline facts: the vitals. The baseline vitals tell you and the reader at what level you found your patient. Is he/she hypotensive, hypertensive, bradycardic, apneic, tachycardiac? The vitals can be used later as an indicator of the direction in which your patient is going (is he or she becoming critical or maintaining?). From here we must document *all* procedures performed and the result. This area, combined with the assessment of your patient, is the most critical legally. Every recognized problem must be documented and treated appropriately (remember that both positive and negative findings must be documented). *Example:* We place a pressure dressing on the distal, inner aspect of the right forearm on our patient to retard the bleeding without losing the pulse. After a few moments the patient complains of a tingling sensation in the fingers on the right side, a reaction that needs to be documented. You loosen the dressing that was applied without an increase of bleeding. Pulse is still present; sensation is now back to the distal region. You have assessed, treated, reassessed, and treated, each time documenting what was found and what was done.

Let's look at each approach discussing the plan within each category. While you read the explanation of each area, turn back to the approach that is being discussed. In this way you will become familiar with each approach and the information at hand. Remember that in each of the following approaches you can use the SOAP or CHARTE format or use the systems approach as a format.

For example, let's look at a predicated scenario applying each of the approaches we have discussed.

> We are called to the scene of an auto accident, where two men are having an argument. While traveling down the highway, one man tries to get out of the car. The driver makes a fast turn, throwing the man out of the car onto the roadway. The driver calls the local emergency number and returns back to the scene. Upon your arrival you see the two men still arguing; one of the men is cradling his left arm with his right arm in sling fashion. You question the patient and assess him, treating the patient in the fashion that you feel is best. Initial vitals: B/P of 134/98, pulse of 120, and respirations of 20 clear bilaterally, equal with good chest expansion. No other injury is observable other than that his left arm has an abrasion across the inner aspect laterally and anteriorly about the shoulders and scapula. A second set of vitals are B/P 128/86, pulse of 100, and respiration of 16. No neurological deficients are found. The patient consents to your treatment. A third set of vitals are B/P of 128/88, pulse of 96, and respirations of 16, still clear bilaterally, equal expansion.

Head-to-Toe Approach

In this category the approach is divided into four basic groups, each group giving you information to be considered. Under observations and special considerations are a list of questions that you may ask yourself or your patient. These questions can also be used in the reassessment process. They are basically a list of considerations. Under history is a list that will give you a start for what has happened, when it happened, and who it happened to. Head-to-toe is the actual assessment of your patient.

Now let's work through our scenario using the category presented. This will give us a chance to become familiar with the material inside.

Under observation we look for bleeding, deformity, discharge, discoloration, tenderness, skin color, and temperature along with a respiratory pattern that we may observe. These problems are points that we must keep in mind during your assessment and reassessment. Special considerations give us the scene setup, what was presented to us as EMS observers. For this example I will use the CHARTE format.

C: The patient was found standing up, arguing with a bystander, deformity of the left arm. Arm cradled by the patient.

You have observed that your patient has a deformity. By noting that the patient was holding his arm and involved in an argument, you establish the consciousness of your patient. Body language is telling you that his arm is hurt.

H: Patient states that he was thrown out of a moving vehicle at approximately 35 mph after leaving a bar down the road approximately 25 minutes ago.

This establishes the condition of your patient neurologically, also the mechanism of injury. The surrounding events are alcohol, possibly masking any other injury. The scene may become dangerous, necessitating rapid removal from the scene, both for scene control and the patient's best interest.

A: Patient alert and oriented to time, person, and place. Alcohol odor present. Pulse equal in the upper extremities, regular at 120. Respirations equal/clear bilaterally with a rate of 20. Blood pressure of 134/98 standing up. Skin color normal, warm/dry. Pupils equal and reactive to light, midpoint. Patient able to move all extremities with the exception of the left arm

Head. No ecchymosis noted, pupils symmetrical with appropriate movement. Face and head symmetrical; no deformity, swelling, discoloration noted. No discharge from ears or nose noted. Minor abrasions about the left occipital region.

Neck. No deformity, discoloration, or swelling noted.

Chest. Normal respiratory pattern, equal expansion, abrasions about the scapula region, all movement symmetrical, no accessory muscle retractions noted, good symmetry and excursion with breathing.

Abdomen. No pain, abrasions, tenderness, guarding, ecchymosis, rigidity noted; abdomen supple in all four quadrants.

Pelvis. Abrasions about the iliac crests and buttocks; no bleeding;

noted pelvic region painful upon palpation when testing for integrity; good pelvic integrity.
Lower Extremities. No pain, discoloration, numbness, deformity, or paralysis noted. Equal pulse; bilaterally, extension and flexation without pain or discomfort. Good capillary refill bilaterally. Patient able to move extremities well within the range of motion.
Upper Extremities. Equal pulse, equal grip strength, good capillary refill, no numbness noted. Deformity, discoloration, swelling, point tenderness of the left distal humerus. Abrasions about the scapula both right and left side and upper posterior thorax.

Here we have assessed our patient from head to toe. Because of the mechanism of injury we wanted to check the patient as much as possible. Basically, we found minor injuries; however, our evaluation was at a level where we were expecting more extensive injuries. We documented all negative and positive findings. The only injury observable was the left arm and the abrasions about the upper torso and hip region. However, by writing down our total evaluation we have stated to the reader beyond a shadow of a doubt the extent of injury found and injuries possible due to the mechanism of injury.

R: Assessment of the patient presented with possible left humerus fracture. Initial vitals: B/P 134/98, pulse of 120, and respirations of 20. Left arm sling and swathe pulse present before and after, good capillary refill before and after splinting. Cervical collar applied with cervical support maintained, patient placed on backboard from an upright position. Cervical immobilization using cervical collar and blanket rolls with tape. Patient strapped to the backboard and placed on ambulance litter. Reassessment of vitals: B/P 128/86 lying down, pulse of 100, respirations 16. Skin warm and dry, pupils equal, and reactive equal grip strength. Patient able to move all extremities upon command, good capillary refill, extension and flexation in all extremities except left arm, due to splint.

Here we state in order the treatment process, the responses to our treatment, with a reassessment component. Note that we stated the position of the patient whenever the vitals were taken.

T: Transported patient to Regional Hospital nonemergency. Advised Emergency Department via cellular phone of patient's condition and treatment priority. Vitals during transport: B/P 128/88, pulse of 96, and respirations 16 supine. Patient remained conscious throughout transportation. Patient turned over to primary trauma nurse at hospital.

Remember that our treatment does not stop at the scene—we still have to reassess and advise the receiving hospital of our patient's condition.

Note: In some areas the system has adopted the latest technology—the cellular phone. This new device is an excellent manner of communication, and if your service has such a capability, you are most fortunate. However, the disadvantage of the cellular phone is that the network does not have EMS priority. Therefore, cellular phones must have a backup system (i.e., radio communications).

E: Patient was found arguing with the driver of the vehicle in which the patient was a passenger. Walking about the accident scene. Patient initially refused treatment and transportation. Patient was advised of the seriousness of the accident. Patient consented to treatment and transportation. Patient requested Regional Hospital.

In exceptions we document all areas, whether or not they have anything to do with the assessment and treatment process because it is information that will help you years from now if there is any question of hospital designation, treatment, alcohol involvement, and so on. For our "story" purpose we had a patient who initially refused treatment and then requested a certain hospital. Later, if a question arises as to whether the hospital was inappropriate, you have documentation which states that it was at the patient's request, the injuries presented were minor, and further-distance hospital would not compromise patient care. The facts become indisputable.

Body Systems Approach

Using this approach, one just finds the system that is most affected, then works through the nine subcategories in order to document what was found. In the scenario given we would turn to the section entitled "The Musculoskeletal System." The written report that we just wrote would be similar using this approach. However, in each subcategory there is the head-to-toe survey. This approach does not use the head-to-toe concept but rather general systems, very much like the nursing concept of documentation discussed earlier.

Here instead of enumerating the head to toe, we would enumerate the system and place the findings within. Again let's use the CHARTE format:

C: Patient involved in auto accident, thrown from a car while traveling approximately 35 mph. Patient found walking about the scene guarding the left arm, cradled with the right arm.

H: Accident occurred approximately 25 minutes ago. Alcohol on breath.

We followed the history section answering all of the questions that apply to this situation.

A: *Pulse.* Equal in all extremities, regular at 120, equal bilaterally with good capillary refill in all extremities. Abrasions about the scapula region, posterior thorax. No lacerations, avulsions noted.
Blood pressure. 134/98 standing upright, right arm.
Respiration. Equal respiratory effort, clear bilaterally. No retractions noted.
Skin color. No cyanosis present, skin warm/dry, redness about the abrasions. Mucous membranes pink.
Pupils. Equal and reactive to light, midpoint equally symmetrical.
Level of consciousness. Patient alert and oriented to person, place, and time. Patient obeys verbal commands.
Ability to move. Good flexation and extension in all extremities.

The rest of the report would look essentially the same. The only element that changes is the assessment.

R: Assessment of the patient presented with possible left humerus fracture. Initial vitals: B/P of 134/98, pulse of 120 and regular, respirations 20 standing upright. Left arm sling and swathe pulse present before and after. Good capillary refill bilaterally. Cervical collar applied with cervical support maintained, patient placed on backboard from an upright position. Cervical immobilization using a cervical collar and blanket roll with tape. Patient strapped to the backboard and placed on ambulance litter. Reassessment vitals: B/P 128/86 in supine position, pulse of 100, and respirations of 16. Patient able to move all extremities upon command, good capillary refill, and flexation good in all extremities except left arm due to splint.

T: Transported patient to Regional Hospital nonemergency. Advised Emergency Department via cellular phone of patient's condition and treatment priority. Vitals during transport: B/P 128/88, pulse 96, and respirations of 16. Patient remained conscious throughout transportation. Patient turned over to primary trauma nurse at hospital.

E: Patient was found arguing with the driver of the vehicle in which patient was a passenger. Patient found walking about the accident scene. Patient initially refused treatment and transportation. Patient was advised of the seriousness of the situation; he then consented to treatment and transportation. Patient requested Regional Hospital.

In some situations the head-to-toe survey works the best; however, it has been my experience that relatively minor conditions follow the systems approach very well. Some students like to use the head-to-toe method as a writing format combining both the head-to-toe information and the body systems approach. This method is extremely helpful when dealing with multiple trauma.

Call Incident Reporting

The third and final approach is organized into categories that best describe the nature of the call. It corresponds to the head-to-toe survey while it hones in on the situation found with all its related problems.

Again I have had students that utilize this approach in combination with the head-to-toe approach. Students and seasoned rescue workers seem to like this category the best. It seems to fit into the rescue worker's frame of thinking.

In this section all one has to do is to find the nature of the situation and follow what is listed, documenting all information that applies to the situation.

C: Patient states that while riding in the automobile, patient fell out of the car, traveling approximately 35 mph. Patient states that he was the passenger and was unrestrained.

H: Accident occurred approximately 25 minutes ago. Patient found walking about scene. Left arm cradled in right arm. Alcohol on breath.

A: Patient alert and oriented to time, person, and place. Alcohol odor present. Pulse equal in all extremities, regular at 120. Good capillary refill in all extremities. Abrasions about the scapula region, posterior thorax, occipital region, and iliac crests/buttocks. No lacerations, avulsions noted. Respiration: equal respiratory effort, clear bilaterally. No retractions noted. Lungs clear bilaterally, rate of 20. Blood pressure of 134/98 standing upright. Skin color pink, warm/dry. Pupils equal and reactive to light, midpoint, equally symmetrical. Patient able to move all extremities with the exception of the left arm.

Head. No ecchymosis noted, pupils symmetrical with appropriate movement. Face and head symmetrical, abrasions about the occipital region. No deformity, swelling, discoloration noted. No discharge from the ears or nose.

Neck. No deformity, discoloration, or swelling noted.

Chest. Normal respiratory pattern, equal, and clear bilaterally, abrasions about the scapula region and posterior thorax. All movement symmetrical, no accessory muscle retractions noted. Good symmetry and excursion with breathing.

Abdomen. No pain, abrasions, tenderness, guarding, ecchymosis, or rigidity noted; abdomen supple.

Pelvis: Abrasions about the iliac crests and buttocks, no bleeding noted, pelvic region painful upon palpation.

Lower extremities. No pain, discoloration, numbness, deformity, or paralysis noted. Equal pulses, extension, and flexation. Good capillary refill. Patient able to move extremities well within the range of motion.

Upper Extremities. Equal pulses, equal grip strength, good capillary refill, no numbness noted. Deformity, discoloration, swelling, point tenderness of the left distal humerus.

R: Assessment of the patient presented with possible left humerus fracture. Initial vitals: B/P of 134/98, pulse of 120, and respirations of 20. Left arm sling and swathe applied, pulse present before and after with good capillary refill. Cervical collar applied with cervical support maintained, patient placed on backboard from an upright position. Cervical immobilization using a cervical collar and blanket roll with tape. Patient strapped to the backboard and placed on ambulance litter. Reassessment vitals: B/P in supine position 128/98, pulse 100, and respirations of 16 clear bilaterally. Patient able to move all extremities upon command, good capillary refill, extension, and flexation in all extremities with the exception of the left arm due to injury and splint.

T: Transported patient to Regional Hospital nonemergency. Advised Emergency Department via cellular phone of patient's condition and treatment priority. Vitals during transport: B/P 128/88, pulse of 96 regular, and respirations of 16. Patient remained conscious throughout transportation. Patient turned over to the primary trauma nurse at the hospital.

E: Patient was found arguing with the driver of the vehicle in which the patient was a passenger. Patient found walking about the accident scene. Patient initially refused treatment and transportation. Patient was advised of the seriousness of the situation, patient consented to treatment and transport (to Regional Hospital only).

As you can see, no two reports are exactly the same; however, to paint the appropriate picture, the same pieces of information must remain the same. The same incident may be recorded in different ways. The main thrust of this book is to organize your thoughts and present them in a meaningful fashion. This kind of organization will help you when dealing with the documentation process. The more you utilize the formats and combine the approaches, the more thorough and skillful you will become in your documentation. Before you know it, you will only need to refer to the book when you are faced with an unusual incident.

In the last example a reference was made to patient refusal. This area is a difficult one to discuss, so I have chosen to talk about it together with other areas that are special in nature. You will find these topics in Chapter 3, "Special Incidents."

Remember that documentation is a skill, and practice makes perfect. You learned to walk by walking, to talk by talking. The more you document, the easier it will become. I trust this book will help you as it has countless others. Good luck!

2

Putting It All Together: Example Reports

The diversity of reports that serve the function of documentation are as many as there are EMS agencies. Some are well done, others are not. All in all, they provide legal representation of the incident. Most of the reports are "fill in the blank" or alphanumeric-type coding. This lends itself to a fairly well organized report and certainly makes it easy from the aspect of what to record. In all of the reports reviewed by this author, it is my opinion that there should be a place for comments. The simple fact of the matter is that no single form can identify all of the possible problems and necessary data points.

In this chapter we look first at data that should be consistently recorded on all EMS reports, then we discuss particular incidents utilizing a generic report. When we look at some reports, the amount of information required by a particular service can be somewhat overwhelming. In the following example reports, we see two entirely different types. Both address the needed information; however, one is "user friendly" (fairly self-explanatory) whereas the other at first glance seems to be confusing. Again, both address the necessary information.

Without getting into specifics, let's look at how we can organize the information. We can look at a report and break it down into three distinct areas for both discussion and quality assurance purposes. The three areas are:

Biographical information
Alarm information
Medical information

Each area has its place, and each is a component of the entire report. If you omit one of these three areas or fill it out partially, you negate the completeness of the report.

The biographical information contains basic general patient identification information: name, date of birth, sex/race, patient weight, physician, incident location, and patient address. Included are the names of agencies and/or units involved, the date, and the names of agencies other than fire or EMS (police, arson investigation, etc.). Some agencies bill for service; in this case additional information is recorded, such as social security numbers, health insurance policy numbers/name of health carrier, and driver's license number or other form of positive identification.

Biographical Information

Name	Age/date of birth	Sex/race
Address of patient	Weight of patient	Private physician
Incident location	Incident date	Map location
Police	Other agencies	Units involved
Social security number	Health insurance number	

The purpose is simple: the report must have an area that properly identifies the person being treated. For agencies in the private sector, for which the service is paid by each person involved, information for the purpose of billing is essential. If money does not come in due to poor report writing, paychecks cannot go out.

The next area is the alarm information, sometimes referred to as alarm history or incident information. This is the place we record information such as incident times: when call was received, time unit enroute to the scene, arrival time at the location, time enroute to the hospital, arrival time at the hospital, and when unit became available for another call; together with the attendants on the scene, mileage to and from the incident, type of call, what hospital the patient went to, and in some cases the person or staff to whom the patient was turned over, extrication time, and support units called in for a specific purpose.

Alarm Information

Incident times
- Call received
- Unit enroute
- Arrive scene
- Arrive patient
- Enroute hospital
- Arrive hospital
- Unit available

Alarm number

Mileage
- To the scene
- To the hospital
- Total mileage

BLS/ALS

Hospital destination

Extrication time

Support units

Attendants
- Rank/badge number
- Organization

Type of incident

Protocol used

This area identifies the alarm history—it is the logistical section of the run report. It is nonspecific as to patient care but identifies required information. Another way of looking at this area is that it helps the administration to identify such things as equipment usage, personnel requirements, and the organizations involved in the incident.

Even though this is basically alarm identification, there are a few points that one must keep in mind when addressing this area. First, it is rare we find the patient waiting for us on the corner or outside the apartment complex. Although the incident took place at a certain location, you may be be required to go to the fourteenth floor. We need to justify the time it took for the rescue crews to make physical contact with the patient. Looking at the report without this information leads to speculation that time was wasted before treatment was begun.

Mileage is an area that is not usually included. We can look at this information from different viewpoints. Administration may need this information from a quality-of-service standpoint. They may want to see how the vehicles are being used. By recording this information, one can look at mileage during both emergency activity and nonemergency activity versus nontransport or emergency utilization activity. Amortization charts can be created for vehicle life spans, giving the manager a solid platform from which he or she can identify and control large vehicle expenditures.

Some services or systems are governed by the medical director or board of medical consortium, in which case basic life support (BLS) versus advanced life support (ALS) units are available. Both the protocol used and the use of a BLS versus an ALS unit is also tracked. Is the appropriate hospital notified, and is that patient delivered to the appropriate hospital? Facility management, protocol identification, and unit utilization, again, are managerial concerns; however, it is our responsibility to supply these data points on a daily basis so as to maintain and improve the quality of service.

Not only does this aid in future management strategies, but it narrows down the incident and draws the picture of what was happening on the scene. Remember that you are constructing a "story" for the reader, drawing a complete and concise picture of what happened at that particular scene.

The final section is the medical information section. It is the actual documentation of the incident from a medical viewpoint. In Chapter 4 we list three separate documentation routes to be used as a reference source when writing an incident medical report. The appendix includes charts and specific information that may be incorporated in the report. In this section we state the problem we were called to, together with what we found in conjunction with treatment modalities.

All three areas of a run report must be completed in an accurate, concise, and logical order. The more organized we are and the neater the handwriting, the more professional the report will look. Take time when writing these reports. They are a reflection of the treatment and the service that your department provided. They are also a reflection of you.

Over the course of my career I have seen some good reports and I have seen some very bad reports. The overall impression of the well-organized, well-written report will communicate to the reader a pride in the work performed as well as the quality and standard of the agency and system.

Some agencies require that all reports be written in black ink, for two reasons. First, when a standard requirement is made department-wide, an overall "look" can be achieved that through standardization of ink and format (remember our format from Chapter 1) will add to the overall presentation if the report goes to court. Second, the report copies more cleanly when a photostat of the report is required.

We are all human and mistakes are going to happen. The run number is going to go where the attendants are supposed to be, and the times are going to be where the incident location is documented. Two problems here: if the report is not turned in, we can neatly rewrite it and only the person who received the report and ourselves are embarrassed. However, if the report is formally turned in, a new report amending the first report, denoting the discrepancy, must be made. Both reports are filed and both will be subpoenaed if the case goes to court. In terms of correcting misspelled words or verbiage that does not make sense, we must cross out the error neatly, using a single line through the middle, and initial the mistake. We do not run a rut in the paper, creating a black hole.

Utilizing the information that we have learned and the reference information provided in Chapter 4 and the appendixes, let's work through a few sample reports. First we work through a report concentrating on the medical section. With each example we work toward completion of the total report. In each scenario a basic guideline is given before the example, thus building the picture we want to provide. Different types of reports are used, enabling you to see how the information can be applied under different circumstances.

Example 1

In this example we use the head-to-toe method and the SOAP format.

A 54-year-old white male has fallen from a tree. He was working at approximately 45 feet. There is an obvious injury to his right femur. He is allergic to penicillin and morphine. He has a history of angina; nitroglycerin is his only medication. He is found on his right side holding his leg. He is conscious. Vitals are as follows: B/P 168/74, P 98, R 24. Second set of vitals: B/P 164/80, P 96, R 22. Third set of vitals: B/P 168/76, P 92, R 22.

S: Patient states that he was working standing on a ladder when he misplaced his footing. Approximate distance was 45 feet to ground. History of angina; medication: nitroglycerin. Allergic to PCN and morphine. C/C right femur pain, and numbness.

O: Pulse is equal in both upper extremities, rate of 98. Respirations are clear bilaterally with a rate of 24, blood pressure is 168/80 partially sitting up. Skin cool/wet and pale. Pupils are equal and reactive, symmetrically. Patient able to move all extremities upon command with the exception of the right leg. Patient alert and oriented to person, place, and time.

Head. Eyes/pupils are equal and reactive to light, pupils are midsize and symmetric, sclera is white and moist. Ears do not show signs of discharge, no ecchymosis noted. Nose is symmetric, no discharge noted. Mouth is symmetric, no cyanosis of the mucosa noted. Head is equal in symmetry; no deformity, discoloration, swelling noted; good facial tone; mental status is alert/oriented to person, place, and time.

Neck. Symmetric; no cyanosis, subcutaneous emphysema, tracheal tugging, or deviation noted. Neck is equal without deformity in the cervical spine area, no discoloration or swelling noted.

Chest. Patient denies pain on inspiration or expiration; however, a grimace of pain is observed upon inspiration. Rate of 24, with equal symmetrical excursion/volume, clear bilaterally. Chest is free of discoloration, swelling, cyanosis, subcutaneous emphysema, and deformity. Good chest integrity without pain upon palpation.

Upper. Equal distal pulses, equal grip strength, skin color/temperature cool/wet, good capillary refill. No paralysis, paresthesia, swelling, discoloration, or deformity noted in the upper extremities.

Abdomen. All four quadrants palpated without pain; no discoloration, swelling cyanosis, guarding, ecchymosis, or pain noted.

Pelvis. Good integrity, abrasions, lacerations about right side, moderate swelling and discoloration, pain upon palpation, strong femoral pulse bilaterally. No deformity noted.

Lower. Numbness, poor capillary refill, shortening with inward rotation, point tenderness, paresthesia, distal pulse not present on right side. Numbness/paresthesia from the mid femur distally, pain upon palpation of the right midshaft femur, deformity, and discoloration of area approximately two times patient's fist. Closed fracture site with poor skin color below site and poor capillary refill distally. Pulse is diminished, associated with distal paresthesia. Left leg is free from injury, good capillary refill, good structure integrity; no deformity, discoloration, or pain noted on left side.

A: Possible fracture of the right femur, with distal pulses diminishing.

P: Initial assessment, maintaining cervical spine support. Oxygen delivered at 15 liters/minute via non-rebreather. Assessment discovered possible right femur fracture with possible blood loss internally. Maintaining cervical support with the application of a cervical collar and manual support. Right femur traction applied manually, patient exhibited some relief, able to place patient supine. New vitals: B/P 164/80, P 96, R 22. Traction splint applied with return of distal pulse, capillary refill improved, numbness/paresthesia relieved. Patient placed on long backboard, cervical immobilization maintained with a blanket roll and tape. Patient secured to spine board. IV established prophylactically D_5W-KVO, 18-gauge left forearm. EKG lead II, sinus rhythm without ectopics. Transported to Regional Hospital without incident. Contacted Regional via Medical Channel 4, advised of patient's condition. Vitals during transport: B/P 168/76, P 92, R 22.

Example 2

Here we use the body systems approach and the SOAP format. (See Figure 2-1.)

We are called to a car versus pedestrian incident; the approximate rate of the vehicle was 45 mph. The patient is a 34-year-old Hispanic female. We observe the patient and notice that she has massive bleeding about the abdomen and left lower extremity deformity. The police on the scene states that after impact, she was thrown approximately 25 feet. Initial vitals: B/P 88/56, P 120, R 24. She is unconscious but responds with incomprehensible words when spoken to. Distal pulses are present; Battle's sign is starting to develop, along with depressed lung sounds on the right side. Second set of vitals: B/P 70/palpation, P 134, R 28 and becoming very shallow. Third set of vitals: B/P 70/palpation, P 136, R 28. Fourth set of vitals: B/P 88/palpation, P 124, R 26.

Example 3

In this example we place emphasis on the medical end associated with advanced life support (ALS) skills. (See Figure 2-2.)

We are called to the home of an elderly black male who has a history of sickle-cell anemia. His wife knows that he takes medication but is not familiar with the type. She does state that they have been a little tight on money lately and she is not sure if he renewed his prescription. The patient is in severe respiratory distress, poor capillary refill, distal pulses present but weak. Lung sounds are distant with mild rales in the bases. Cyanosis is severe and quite obvious even though the patient has a fairly dark complexion. Once you start to transport the patient, he degrades into ventricullar fibrillation. Initial vitals are B/P 90/46, P 126, R 38. Second set of vitals reveals a decompensation to B/P 56/palpation, P 146, R 44 shallow. Third set indicates cardiac arrest with agonal respirations.

Example 4

In this case we use a combination of the call incident report writing method and the head-to-toe method. We use the CHARTE format. (See Figure 2-3.)

A 23-year-old female is shot with a .38 caliber hand gun at point-blank range. She is conscious and alert, understands all that is going on, and appears to be healthy. She is found in the bedroom of her apartment, stating that she has been raped. She is very anxious and nervous at EMS arrival. Vitals are B/P 100/78, P 118, R 22. After a short time she becomes unresponsive and a drop in vitals are noticed. B/P 78/palpation, P 128, R 32. The entrance wound is in the upper right quadrant with an exit wound in the lower posterior thoarax. Third set of vitals: 78/palpation, P 128, R 32.

Example 5

Here we use the call incident approach again. This case is a type that you will experience often—it is a recurrent scenario. (See Figure 2-4.)

We are called to a man down in the park. Upon arrival we are greeted by law enforcement personnel stating that they tried to wake this man two hours ago. You find a transient, strong smell of alcohol. You attempt to wake him and do so.

Example 6

In this example we use the body systems approach and the CHARTE format. (See Figure 2-5.)

Your unit is called to the corner of First and Main. The police have detained a man with blood about his face and vomiting. Patient is somewhat violent, however will talk to you; eventually, he becomes unresponsive. While able to verbalize the patient tells you that he fell out of a car while driving at a high rate of speed. Patient states that his head hit something hard on impact. You notice that the left side and occipital region are severely deformed, with blood coming from the nose and ears. Initial vitals are B/P 180/120, P 88, R 30. During immobilization patient becomes unconscious; vitals are B/P 210/128, P 66, R 10. The third and fourth set of vitals are the same as the second set.

PINELLAS COUNTY EMS REPORT

FDID | Incident No. 02 | FEDERAL TAX #59-6000800 | MEDICARE #A0601 | Mo. 5 | Day 11 | Year 98 | Casualty No. 1 of 1

Race: [ ] 1-White [ ] 2-Black [✓] 3-Hispanic [ ] 4-Asian [ ] 5-Amer. Indian / Alaskan Native | Sex (M (F)) | Unit - Sta.- Shift: 01, R, 1, C

Last Name: HISPANIC | First Name: FEMALE | M.I. | D.O.B.: 5-11-64 | Age: 34 | Home Phone: —

Address of Incident: HIGHWAY 30 AND STATE ROAD 130

CHIEF COMPLAINT: AUTO VS PEDESTRIAN

HOW/WHERE FOUND: IN INTERSECTION Ⓡ LATERAL RECUMBENT

MEDICAL HISTORY: AUTO VS PEDESTRIAN AT 45mph

CURRENT MEDS.: UNKNOWN – NONE FOUND ON PATIENT – NO ID FOUND

ALLERGIES: NKA

PHYSICIAN: UNKNOWN

INITIAL ASSESSMENT

L.O.C: INCOMP. WORDS | Coma Sc.: 3

SKIN: COOL/MOIST | Trauma Sc.: 8

LUNG SOUNDS: DEPRESSED Ⓡ

PUPILS: TIME 1802 REACTION SLOW/SLUGGISH

MID POINT

VITAL SIGNS:

Time	B/P	Pulse	Resp.	ID #
1803	88/56	120	24	OA
1808	70/pal	134	28	OA
1809	70/pal	136	28	OB
1818	88/pal	124	26	OA

Time	Procedure	Dose/Route	ID Number
1803	Assessment	Vitals	OA
1804	C-spine support	C-collar	OB
1804	O_2	15L/min MASK	OB
1805	Monitor	Lead II S.Tach	OA
1806	IV-RL open	16 Ⓛ AC	OA
1808	MAST-legs only	Inflated	OA
1808	Re-assessment	Vitals	OB
1808	Placed on LBB		OA
1809	Re-assessment	Vitals	OA
1810	Load pt into amb		OB/OA
1810	Enroute hosp.		
1811	Hosp. Contacted via Radio		
1818	Reassessment	Vitals	
1822	Arrive Hosp.		
1825	TOT staff		

REMARKS (SOAP) S: Pt found in roadway at 30+SR130; Ⓡ lateral recumbent position. Pt unconscious. No ID found. Pt was struck while crossing street, per bystanders car traveling approx. 45mph. O: Pules present in all extremities, delayed capillary refill, Pulse as stated, BP equal in both arms. Respiratory effort equal with depressed sounds on Ⓡ side, No tracheal tugging, Nasal flaring or diaphragmatic breathing noted. Battle's sign developing, sudden/slow resp. starting to develop. Volume of breath depressed. Pt unconscious – incomprehensible words when spoken to. HEAD – Pupils mid-point slow to reaction, symmetric, sclera white/moist. Ears show no signs of discharge however battle's sign becoming worse. Mucosa slightly cyanotic, No deformity/swelling noted about the head NECK — Symmetrical no cyanosis, without deformity. No tracheal

Reported by Crew: A. PARAMEDIC, B. EMT

Rec. Phy. ______ Tele. Phy. ______ Reviewed by ______ Medical Dir. ______

Hospital Contacted	Transport to	Transport by	Grid
10	10	06	0102

Alarm Time	Arrival First	Arrival ALS	Arrival AMB	Transport Time	Time In Service	Situation Found	Action Taken
1800	1803	1803	1804	1810	1830	423	206

FIRST RESPONDER COPY

FIGURE 2-1

TRANSPORT	FDID	Incident No.	Unit

REMARKS (SOAP) tugging noted. CHEST – Ⓡ side lung sound depression – equal excursion, symmetry chest is free of discoloration, swelling, or cyanosis/subcutaneous emphysema. Good chest integrity. ABDOMEN – LLQ 2-4 inch deep laceration – extensive external bleeding = Abdomen is discolored, cyanotic with swelling and organ protruding at the laceration site. PELVIS – Good integrity. Free from abrasions, lacerations deformity, swelling. LOWER EXT – Ⓛ lower extremity deformity. Poss closed tibia and fibula fracture. Distal pulse present. Capillary refill delayed. Ⓡ extremity is unremarkable UPPER EXT – No deformity, discoloration, swelling or cyanosis noted pulse present bilaterally with delayed capillary refill. A: Possible Ⓡ pneumothorax Ⓛ eviscerated abdomen and possible Ⓛ tibia/fibula fracture. P: SEE TIME LINE ON PAGE ONE. transported to Ocean Memorial with paramedic accomp.

Review Request

Reported by ______	Rec. Phy. ______
Crew ______	Tele. Phy. ______
______	Reviewed by ______
______	Medical Dir. ______

PATIENT REFUSAL

I hereby certify that I refuse ALL TREATMENT [ ] by the Emergency Medical Services for myself (my son [ ] my daughter [ ] my wife [ ] other [ ]), and/or refuse transportation to the closest or most advisable health care facility, and insist that transport be to ______ for my own reasons, notwithstanding that such treatment and/or recommended transport may be deemed necessary to preserve life or promote recovery, and that I have been so advised by the Emergency Medical Services Personnel. I (we) hereby accept all responsibility connected with action and hereby release the Emergency Medical Service, its Paramedics, and Pinellas County, its officers and agents from any and all liability and responsibility whatsoever for any untoward results due to my (our) refusal of such treatment and/or recommended transport against the advice and urging of the said Paramedics.

Patient or Authorized Agent or Guardian ______ Witness ______

PATIENT AUTHORIZATION

I, the undersigned, hereby authorize directly to Sunstar, benefits otherwise payable to me but not to exceed regular charges for this type of service. If I am entitled to Medicare benefits, I authorize any holder of medical or other information about me to release to Social Security Administration or its intermediaries or carriers, any information needed for this or related Medicare claim. I permit a copy of this authorization to be used in place of the original, and request payment of medical insurance benefits either to myself or to Sunstar. I understand I am financially responsible to Sunstar for charges not covered by this authorization and do hereby guarantee payment of this bill within thirty (30) days. I further agree that if collection is made by suit or otherwise, I agree to pay all collection costs including a reasonable attorney's fee. I hereby approve release of information pertinent to hospital confinement, doctor's treatment, and diagnosis for claims for insurance benefits. I have been advised that I may be responsible for any unpaid portion of these charges not covered by insurance.

Signed X ______ Patient or Policyholder

Guarantor's Last Name	First Name	MI	Phone	SSN
				— —

Guarantor's Address

Patient's Last Name	First Name	MI	D.O.B.	Sex	SSN
					— —

Start Miles	End Miles	Total Miles	Oxygen	Waiting Time
.	.	.		

[ ] Private No. Ins. [ ] Private Ins. [ ] Worker's Comp

[ ] Medicare [ ] Medicaid [ ] V.A.

[ ] Membership [ ] Other ______

Number ______

Place of Employment

Address

Diagnosis	Diagnosis	Diagnosis	Diagnosis	Diagnosis

FIRST RESPONDER COPY

FIGURE 2-1 *continued*

1. PATIENT'S NAME	2 SEX	3. DOB or AGE	4 RACE	5. WT./KG	6. RES.	PRIVATE PHYSICIAN
ELDERLY, BLACK MALE	M	020636	B	85kg	Y	Dr. Nice

7. PATIENT'S ADDRESS	8. RUN NUMBER	9.	10 AGY	11. STN	UNIT	DEST DET
121 E. First St.	02020	1	K	99	199	D

12. INCIDENT LOCATION	13. RUN DATE	14. S.T.R	15 DUP	POLICE
121 E. First St.	041694	222340	Y	NONE

16. CALL REC'D	0926	23. MILEAGE		24 TYPE OF CALL	A
17. UNIT ENRT	0926	TO 1.1		25. DISP. OF CALL	B
18. ARR'VD LOC	0930	FROM 2.6		26. PT TAKEN TO	N
19. ARR'VD PT	0931	TOTAL 3.7		27. EXTRICATION	—
20. PT DEP'D	0946	39. ALS Y		28. SEAT BELT	—
21. ARR'VD DEST	1005	40. ARRHYTHMIA 2		29. CHILD RESTR.	—
22. UNIT AVAIL.	1006			30. HELMET	—
				31. ANATOMY OF INJ.	—
				32 GLASGOW COMA SCORE	12

33. NATURE OF RUN: T

34. PROTOCOL USED: G

ALLERGIES: NKA

REPORT RECEIVED

PHYSICIAN'S SIGNATURE

35. ATTENDANT A	A. PARAMEDIC	OC	4336
36. ATTENDANT B	B PARAMEDIC	OC	ST911
37. OTHER O	Eng. Comp. 39		
38. OTHER O			

**BEAR DOWN WHILE WRITING
ALL COPIES MUST BE LEGIBLE**

COMMENTS: C: Pt states progressive dyspnea since last night which has become worse H: Sickle Cell anemia. Pt is on medication unknown type - has not been taking do to lack of income A: Pt was sleeping at the start of the event, pt is now in livingroom sitting in chair. Pulse is weak/thready, Resp. shallow clear bilaterally, distal grip equal in upper extremites with pain - General full body pain upon movement. Distal pulse present in all extremities with poor capillary refill. Severe cyanosis about the mucosa. Since start of exam pt's sensorium has decreased. R: SEE TIME LINE BELOW

TIME	L.O.C.	B.P.	P	R	CC/EKG	TREATMENT	RESPONSE	AID/ATT
0931	3	90/46	126	38		Assessment	Vitals - Hx	S/A
0932						O2 - Non Rebreather	15L/min - mucosa	/
						cyanotic, Mental status decreasing - Pt		/
						supine high trendeleburg position.		/
0933					S. TACH	Monitor Lead II		P/A
0934		90/46	130	38		IV D5W - KVO 18g (L) Forehand blood drawn		A/B
0941						Pt placed on amb litter - Mental status		/
						decrease to incomprehensible words,		/
						cyanosis increase, Supine position		/
0942	1	56/pal	146	44		Reassessment - High Trendeleburg to		S/A
						supine B/V/M over-ride / Hyperventilate		P/B

SIGNATURE: A Paramedic DATE: 4/16/94

40-1 (8/88) ORANGE COUNTY, FLORIDA, EMS

FIGURE 2-2

Page 2 of 2
(cont.)

1. PATIENT'S NAME
ELDERLY BLACK MALE

7. PATIENT'S ADDRESS
121 E. First St

8. RUN NUMBER
002020

12. INCIDENT LOCATION
121 E. First St

13. RUN DATE
041694

TIME	L.O.C.	B.P.	P	R	EKG	INTERVENTION	RESPONSE	ATT
0946						Load Pt in Amb		
0946						Enroute Regional Hospital		
0948		0/0	0	0	V. Fib	Re-assessment	Cardiopulmonary Arrest	4/A
0948						CPR	Pulse with compression	4/A
0949						Defibrillate @200 w/s	Ventricular Fib	7/B
0950						Defibrillate @300 w/s	Ventricular Fib	7/B
0951						Defibrillate @360 w/s	Ventricular Fib	7/B
0952						Epinephrine 1:10,000	1mg IVP EMD	A/A
0954						ETT—cord visual, equal	breath sounds #8.0	E/A
						good chest rise with improved color		
0953						BVM with ETT	Hypervent.	X/A
0955					EMD	Fluid Challenge	200ml RL	Y/B
0957		56/pal	100	0		Pulse regained—cap-refill delayed, lungs		
						clear, assist ventilations with BVM		4/A
1002						Dopamine 400mg in 250ml for 5mcg/kg/min		9/A
						infused at 16 mcg/min		
1000						Regional contacted via Medical Radio		

COMMENTS: T: Transport to Regional with Fire-Medic aboard AMB - Pt lost pulse and respirations during transport phase with successful pulse and Blood pressure response. B/P, P, R taken just prior to arrival at hosp. B/P - 90/46, Pulse 100, R-0 ASSISTED. Turned patient over to ED nurse.

SIGNATURE: A Paramedic DATE: 4/16/94

40-1 (6/87) ORANGE COUNTY, FLORIDA, EMS

FIGURE 2-2 *continued*

INDIAN RIVER COUNTY EMERGENCY MEDICAL SERVICES
RUN REPORT

DATE: 9-1-60

PATIENT'S NAME: Young Female AGE: 23 D.O.B. 12-2-37 SEX: F RACE: C

INCIDENT ADDRESS: 333 EAST 6th

HOME ADDRESS: 333 EAST 6th SS#

CHIEF COMPLAINT: GSW URQ – SEXUAL ASSAULT Approx 30 min ago / found in bedroom

MEDICATIONS: None

ALLERGIES: NKA DR.

ADDITIONAL Hx: None

COMMENTS: C: Pt states she was raped by her boyfriend then shot by another man – pt found supine on bed, clothes partially on with lower torso wrapped in the sheets. Significant blood loss noted in the sheets H: Police state pt was shot with a .38 caliber hand gun at point blank range Police advise pt has become increasingly nervous since our arrival A: Pt A/OX3, Skin cool/clammy, PEARL, Lungs Clear bilaterally with pain upon inspiration on the Ⓡ side, Sensorium is normal and understands all that is going on around her. Capillary Refill is normal, able to move all extremities. Distal Pulse present in all extremities, good Flex/Extension in lower, good-grip good in upper extrem. Entrance wound noted URQ with Exit lower posterior thorax with fair resp. status.

PRIORITY 1-2-③ CONDITION: GOOD ☐ FAIR ☐ SERIOUS ☑ CRITICAL ☐

TIMES REC: 1000 10-8 1001 10-97 1005 10-51 ER 10-6 ER 10-98

VITAL SIGNS:	Time	BP	P	R	EKG
#1 Time	1005	100/78	118	22	S. TACH
#2 Time		78/pal	128	32	S. TACH
#3 Time		78/pal	128	32	S. TACH
#4 Time					

FIGURE 2-3

EXAM	NORMAL	ABNORMAL	EXAM COMMENTS
HEAD	☑	☐	No fluid from ears, nose or mouth—noted
EYES	☑	☐	Pearl—equal reation midpoint
EARS	☑	☐	No fluid
NOSE	☑	☐	No fluid
MOUTH	☑	☐	Teeth intacted—good color of mucosa
NECK	☑	☐	Normal without deformity
CHEST WALL	☑	☑	Clear bilaterally with pain on inspiration Ⓡ exit
LUNGS	☑	☐	wound noted lower posterior does not seem to be
HEART	☑	☐	compromising Cardio Resp.
ABDOMEN	☑	☑	URQ Entrance wound point blank .38 powder burns
M/F ORGANS	☑	☐	No discharge noted
ARMS	☑	☐	Equal grip—good capillary refill
LEGS	☑	☐	Full range of motion—good capillary refill
BACK	☑	☐	
NEURO	☑	☐	Feels full sensation in all extrem. and along lateral
SKIN	☐	☑	body—Skin cool/clammy

ORDERS BY DR. ☑ PROTOCOL

TIME:	IV#1- RL	FLOW- KVO	SITE- Ⓛ AC	SIZE- 14g	#ATTEMPTS- 1
TIME:	IV#2-	FLOW-	SITE-	SIZE-	#ATTEMPTS-
TIME:	MED-	DOSE-	ROUTE-	RESULTS-	
TIME:	MED-	DOSE-	ROUTE-	RESULTS-	
TIME:	MED-	DOSE-	ROUTE-	RESULTS-	
TIME:	MED-	DOSE-	ROUTE-	RESULTS-	
TIME:	MED-	DOSE-	ROUTE-	RESULTS-	

SPLINTS/DRESSINGS: MAST APPLIED, Pt Placed on backboard—Legs section only inflate.

TYPE CALL: ALS ☑ BLS ☐ CANCELLED ☐ REFUSAL ☐ SIG7 ☐

HOSPITAL: I.R.M.H. ☐ HUMANA ☐ OTHER ☑

TRANSPORTATION: FELLSMERE ☐ I.R.S.P.S. ☐ SEBASTIAN ☐ I.R.C.F.D. ☐ I.R.C. EMS. ☐ OTHER ☐

FIRE - UNIT # PERSONNEL: A Paramedic, B Paramedic

AMB - UNIT # PERSONNEL: PARA. JO Paramedic DR. FA. EMT.

DATE:	CARDIAC ____ ARREST ____ OD ____ SIG4 ____
DISPATCH #:	RESP. ____ SEIZURE ____ ABD ____ TRAUMA ✓
PROVIDER #: MAP ZONE #:	DIABETIC ____ SPINAL ____ CVA ____ OTHER ____
RESPONDING FROM:	SIGNATURE: A Paramedic

WHITE—ALS YELLOW—BILLING PINK—AMB GOLDENROD—HOSPITAL

FIGURE 2-3 *continued*

PINELLAS COUNTY EMS REPORT

FDID | Incident No. 011 | FEDERAL TAX #59-6000800 | MEDICARE #A0601 | Mo. 3 | Day 6 | Year 90 | Casualty No. 1 of 1

Race [✓] 1-White [ ] 2-Black [ ] 3-Hispanic [ ] 4-Asian [ ] 5-Amer. Indian / Alaskan Native | Sex (M F) — M | Unit - Sta.- Shift: 01 01 B

Last Name: JOE | First Name: LOST | M.I. | D.O.B. 12-6-40 | Age 30 | Home Phone —

Address of Incident: EAST AND SOUTH AVE

CHIEF COMPLAINT: Police found pt sleeping

HOW/WHERE FOUND: bench on side of road

MEDICAL HISTORY: None

CURRENT MEDS.: None

ALLERGIES: NKA

PHYSICIAN:

Time	Procedure	Dose/Route	ID Number
2212	Assessment	Vitals	OA
2219	Medical Release Signed Police witnessed		OB

INITIAL ASSESSMENT

L.O.C — 0 — Coma Sc.

SKIN warm/dry Trauma Sc.

LUNG SOUNDS

PUPILS : TIME REACTION

VITAL SIGNS:

Time	B/P	Pulse	Resp.	ID #
2212	124/86	88	12	OA

REMARKS (SOAP) S: Pt found by Police sleeping on bench. Unable to wake EMS called. O: Pt sleeping with strong odor of EtOH, Pt seems not to be in any distress. Observation skin warm/dry with good capillary refill, lungs clear posteriorly. After repeated attempts at waking this person, Pt opens eyes and sits up. Pt advises us he is all right that he was "just sleeping it off". Pt answers all questions Pt A/Ox3 strong EtOH consumption. Pt refuses and signs medical release.

Reported by: A. Paramedic

Crew: B. Paramedic

Rec. Phy.

Tele. Phy.

Reviewed by

Medical Dir.

Hospital Contacted	Transport to	Transport by	Grid

Alarm Time	Arrival First	Arrival ALS	Arrival AMB	Transport Time	Time In Service	Situation Found	Action Taken
2210	2212	2214	2215				

FIRST RESPONDER COPY

FIGURE 2-4

TRANSPORT	FDID	Incident No.	Unit

REMARKS (SOAP) ______

Review Request

Reported by	A Paramedic	Rec. Phy.	
Crew	B Paramedic	Tele. Phy.	
		Reviewed by	
		Medical Dir.	

PATIENT REFUSAL

I hereby certify that I refuse ALL TREATMENT [ ] by the Emergency Medical Services for myself (my son [ ] my daughter [ ] my wife [ ] other [ ]), and/or refuse transportation to the closest or most advisable health care facility, and insist that transport be to ______ for my own reasons, notwithstanding that such treatment and/or recommended transport may be deemed necessary to preserve life or promote recovery, and that I have been so advised by the Emergency Medical Services Personnel. I (we) hereby accept all responsibility connected with action and hereby release the Emergency Medical Service, its Paramedics, and Pinellas County, its officers and agents from any and all liability and responsibility whatsoever for any untoward results due to my (our) refusal of such treatment and/or recommended transport against the advice and urging of the said Paramedics.

Patient or Authorized Agent or Guardian [signature] Witness Police 107 #6

PATIENT AUTHORIZATION

I, the undersigned, hereby authorize directly to Sunstar, benefits otherwise payable to me but not to exceed regular charges for this type of service. If I am entitled to Medicare benefits, I authorize any holder of medical or other information about me to release to Social Security Administration or its intermediaries or carriers, any information needed for this or related Medicare claim. I permit a copy of this authorization to be used in place of the original, and request payment of medical insurance benefits either to myself or to Sunstar. I understand I am financially responsible to Sunstar for charges not covered by this authorization and do hereby guarantee payment of this bill within thirty (30) days. I further agree that if collection is made by suit or otherwise, I agree to pay all collection costs including a reasonable attorney's fee. I hereby approve release of information pertinent to hospital confinement, doctor's treatment, and diagnosis for claims for insurance benefits. I have been advised that I may be responsible for any unpaid portion of these charges not covered by insurance.

Signed X ______ Patient or Policyholder

Guarantor's Last Name	First Name	MI	Phone	SSN
				– –

Guarantor's Address

Patient's Last Name	First Name	MI	D.O.B.	Sex	SSN
LOST	JOE		12/6/40	M	– –

[ ] Private No. Ins. [ ] Private Ins. [ ] Worker's Comp

[ ] Medicare [ ] Medicaid [ ] V.A.

[ ] Membership [ ] Other ______

Number ______

Start Miles	End Miles	Total Miles	Oxygen	Waiting Time
.	.	.		

Place of Employment

Address

Diagnosis	Diagnosis	Diagnosis	Diagnosis	Diagnosis

FIRST RESPONDER COPY

FIGURE 2-4 *continued*

History:

MARY, SCOTT
Patient's Name

Age: 41 **Sex** [x] Male [ ] Female **Race:** [x] Asian [ ] Black [ ] White [ ] Other ______

Arrival: [ ] W/C [ ] Ambulatory [ ] Stretcher [x] Ambulance [ ] Helicopter [ ] Other ______ **Dr.** ______

Chief Complaint: "Fell out of car while driving at high rate of speed"

P.I: Left side occipital region - severely deformed with blood coming from the nose and ears. Pt is conscious but slips into an unresponsive state from time to time. Pt found on side of road lying in a semi-recumbant position.

(Location, Quality, Intensity, Quantity, Cronology, Setting, Scenario of First Symptoms, Aggravation and Alleviation, Associated Complaints, Attempts to Modify)

P.M.I:

General state of health GOOD

Past illnesses: [ ] Heart Disease [ ] Emphysema [ ] Asthma [ ] Diabetes [ ] Ulcers [ ] Hypertension [ ] Cancer [ ] Other } UNKNOWN

Hospitalizations (include psychiatric illnesses): Poss. Psy Hx - Rx - Lithium

Surgery: UNKNOWN

Allergies: NKA
Include environmental, ingestible or drug related!

Immunizations: ______

Substance Abuse (include alcohol, cigarettes, and street drugs: Poss. EtOH

Medications (include over the counter meds): Lithium

Mental: [x] Conscious [x] Unconscious [ ] Alert [ ] Oriented { Person [ ] Place [ ] Time [ ]

Status: [ ] Restless [x] Combative [ ] Co-operative [ ] Other ______

Skin: [ ] Warm [ ] Dry [x] Cool [x] Clammy [ ] Mottled [x] Cyanotic [x] Diaphoretic [ ] Jaundice [ ] Flushed [ ] Pallor [ ] Pink [x] Other Cyanosis about mucosa

Pupils: [ ] PEARL [x] Other (L) Dilated **Visual Acuity:** OD [/] OS [/]

Skull: (L) scapula - deformity
(Describe)

ENT: [x] Draining [ ] Post Nasal [ ] Difficulty swallowing [x] Other BLOOD and Poss. CSF

Face: CLEAR
(Describe)

FIGURE 2-5

Neck: ☑ Supple ☐ Engorged Veins ☐ Nuchal Rigidity ☐ Other ______

Chest:
Heart Sounds: NORMAL
Lungs: ☑ Clear ☐ Rales ☐ Rhonchi ☐ Other
Resp: ☑ Shallow ☑ Labored ☐ Retraction ☑ Deep ☐ SOB ☐ Injury ☑ Slow ☐ Effortless ☐ Rapid ☐ Kussmaul Rate ____

Abdomen:
☑ Soft ☐ Rebound ☐ Distended ☐ Guarding ☐ Rigid ☐ Nausea ☐ Swollen ☐ Emesis
UL UR LL LR
√ Bowel Sounds
unremarkable

G.U: ☐ Burning ☐ Urgency ☐ Color ______ ☐ Frequency ☐ Hematuria ☐ Other ______

GYN:
☐ Bleeding Discharge ☐ LMP ☐ Para ☐ Gravida ☐ Ab
MALE
(State "Male" if so)

Spine: unremarkable (Describe)

Extremity:
Injury: None Pulses: Equal
☐ Warm ☑ Cyanotic ☐ Pink ☐ Mottled ☑ Cool ☐ Edema
☑ Weakness ☑ Movement
(R) sided weakness at times

Vital Signs:

Time	2210	2215	2220	2225		
Sys / Di	180/120	210/128	210/128	210/128		
Pulse	88	66	106	66		
Resp	30	10	10	10		
Temp.						

Cardiac Monitor EKG: S. Rhy. → S. Brady.

Your Tentative Diagnosis: Skull fracture

Expected Treatment: C/O, C-SPINE support, LBB, IV, TRANSPORT ASAP

Actual Diagnosis (ask Dr.): Depressed skull fracture

Actual Treatment (list all lab work, x-rays, Iv, meds, etc.) ______

A Paramedic
Signature

9/6/90
Date

FIGURE 2-5 *continued*

Clinical Narrative

Date: 9/6/90 **Location:** MAIN/FIRST

Clinical: Poss. Skull fracture

C: Pt. stated he was thrown/fell out of a car, traveling at a high rate of speed. Pt goes between unconsciousness and consciousness with episodes of violent behavior. Pt found on side of the road with police detaining pt. Blood about the face.

H: History is undetermined - Poss Psychiatric Hx. Lithium Medication bottle found by police in Ⓛ pants pocket. Pt unable or will not tell us of any history.

A: Pt when conscious is A/OX3 able to respond to all verbal commands with approp. action. Episodes of violent behavior and episodes of unconsciousness. Bystanders state that he was noticed approx. 45min ago, however EMS was not called ~~unit~~ until 15min ago.

HEAD: Pt has deformity of the occipital region, blood/CSF from the ears and nose. Blood about the face - Depressed region of the skull - occipital area.

NECK: Unremarkable, supple, No JVD noted. Cynosis not present.

CHEST: Good chest integrity, Lung sounds clear bital. Breath sounds shallow/labored when uncons. Deep and slow when conscious. No deformity, discoloration, swelling or ecchmosis noted.

ABD: All four quad's supple, without discoloration, deformity or pain.

LOWER EXT: Pt able to move when conscious. Starts to posture when unconscious. Good pedial pulse, Good Cap-Refill, extend/flex. when conscious. No deformity, discoloration, swelling noted.

UPPER EXT: Pt able to move when conscious. Starts to posture when unconscious. Good pedial pulse. Good Cap-Refill. Good grip strength. No deformity, discoloration or swelling noted.

R: Upon arrival maintained cervical support. Pt placed on O_2 non-rebreather at 15L/min. Pt's mucosa pink and remained pink throughout event. Good capillary refill before and after O_2.

FIGURE 2-5 *continued*

Clinical Narrative

Date: 9/6/90 **Location:** MAIN/FIRST

Clinical: Poss. Skull fracture

Cervical Collar applied and C-spine maintained. IV D5W-KVO
(L) AC with 18g. Pt log-rolled onto longbackboard and
secured with T-bandages, C-collar applied, Cervical Immob.
device. Monitor shows Normal Sinus to Tachycardia
without ectopics. Pt reassessed every 5min. Hospital
contacted via cellular phone.

T: Transported via Rescue to Hospital. Pt on backboard
CID, C-collar in place. O_2 maintained at 15L/min
Monitor NSR → ST → NSR. Mucosa/Capillary Refill
Pink throughout incident. Resp. status maintained by
pt. TOT Hosp. upon arrival without delay.

E: Pt found detained by police in supine position.

FIGURE 2-5 *continued*

3

Special Incident Report Writing

Patient Refusal

Patient refusal seems to be the one area that health care professionals have a problem with. I think in the back of our minds it is very hard to realize that someone could be refusing our services. In reality, they are not truly refusing your service—they have nothing against you personally. They are refusing the service as a whole, the system as a whole. By documenting this you are saying that this person is refusing the service against your better judgment. Your judgment is a combination of your training, continuing education, and experience as a health care professional.

It is important to have a record of everything that happened on the scene. I have been asked in the past how much you should document. The answer is: as much as possible. The problem lies with how much is too much. My suggestion is to approach the situation as if you were going to treat this person. Give him or her a full objective and subjective head-to-toe survey. Then write it down in a logical, concise manner. If the patient states that he or she feels that your procedures are unnecessary, state on your run report that you offered field evaluation but the patient refused. Notation of refusal of service is extremely important. It is truly unfortunate that we have become such a legalistic society, one in which most people believe that all disputes must be handled through legal channels. This is especially unfortunate when we are dealing with human life in an emergency situation. Whatever your personal thoughts on the subject, we have to accept the reality of litigation and protect ourselves accordingly.

Depending on whom you speak with, patient refusal may not weigh heavily in a situation. However, the legal system looks at it quite differently. By stating on paper what went on, what you did, and what the patient said, you can re-create the circumstances in question and justify all actions taken.

How do we document such a mess? As stated in Chapter 2, gather as much information as you possibly can: name, age, address, and so on. As you are asking for information (for your report), start injecting some subjective questioning. Ask why they do not want to go to the hospital, and be cognizant of the patient's needs: "The ambulance costs too much"; "I'm afraid of rescue trucks." If your patient truly does not want your service, but you feel that it is in the best interest for your patient to go to the hospital, be sure to document thoroughly. Ask if you can give him or her a cursory medical evaluation, take vitals, ask questions as to how the situation developed, what precipitated the event, who was involved, and why the person refuses to be transported or/and why cursory examination/evaluation is being refused.

Investigating how we would document such a situation:

> If your patient will allow you to perform a cursory medical exam, evaluate the person as much as you can. In essence you are giving him or her a secondary survey. Ask questions and record your run report as designated in Chapter 2. Use a format and stick to it. Write down all information that you elicit from the patient.

Looking at two examples:

Example 1. You are called to the local grocery store, man fallen. Upon arrival the assistant manager meets you at the door. He states that this man came into the store and fell in the produce department. You ask where the patient is and he directs you to the manager's office, where the patient is sitting in a chair and the manager is making out an incident report. You walk in and start questioning your patient.

First, look at the set of circumstances as stated by the manager's assistant: the person fell in the produce department. Do not question the manager or his assistant. Wait until you can communicate directly with the patient.

You question the patient and the patient states that he slipped on a wet spot. You ask the patient how he got from the produce area to the office. You ask the manager (not the assistant) if there was a wet spot. The manager responds: "not to the best of my knowledge." Your patient becomes very frustrated and starts to yell at the manager that he is going to sue, stating that the assistant manager helped him to the office.

Now look at what we have walked into: a possible lawsuit in which you are not directly involved; however, your actions can and will direct the outcome of the case if it goes into a courtroom. Inadvertently, your department, city, and service as well as yourself become very much involved.

You question the patient starting with preliminary information: name, age, medical history, medications, and so on. You find that your patient does not have a history, is elderly, possibly on Medicare, and takes no medication. Your patient is moving about; he does not state that anything is hurt.

Document this utilizing the musculoskeletal section in the system approach with SOAP as the format.

S: Patient states that while shopping, he slipped on a wet spot in the produce section of the store. He was then helped to his feet by other patrons and directed to the manager's office. Patient was able to walk there with some help from the assistant manager. Patient is not on any medications, has no medical history, and is not complaining of any pain.

By stating exactly what happened and why/who got him up, the liability for medical problems rests on the store.

O: Patient is a 72-year-old male, alert, and oriented to time, person, and place. States that he is healthy and does not have a medical history. Patient was found sitting in an office chair. Accident occurred approximately 25 minutes ago. Pulse is 88 equal in all extremities, regular and strong. Respirations are 18 clear bilateral, equal excursion, and symmetric blood pressure of 146/98. Head is unremarkable, equal symmetry, no fluid from the ears or nose noted. Neck is unremarkable. Chest is unremarkable with equal bilateral breath sounds. Skin is pink, warm, and dry. Pupils are equal and reactive to light. Equal grip strength, equal pulses, equal flexation and extension in the upper extremities. Lower extremities: nothing remarkable, equal pulses distally, equal flexation and extension. No deformity or discoloration; pain upon palpation noted throughout entire survey. Patient is alert and oriented to person, place, and time.

A: Patient states that he does not feel any pain in any particular area but has full body discomfort. Refuses medical treatment and transportation to the hospital.

P: Patient is again advised that he should go to the hospital for further medical evaluation, as our evaluation is not complete. Patient refuses treatment and transportation. We again state that it is in his best interest to be evaluted by a physician. Patient refuses. Patient is alerted to the possibility of either a fracture or other internal injuries. Patient refuses treatment and transport. Report is signed, witnessed by the store manager and a police officer.

By stating the procedures followed, requesting three times that the patient go to the hospital, and giving the patient the opportunity to evaluate the situation, you have placed the liability on the patient and the store. The patient was advised of the situation, understood the situation, and knew what the consequences were. You were there simply to provide medical assistance, which was refused. Whenever you have a refusal, if possible have a police officer witness the document, adding his or her badge number, department, and rank. If this case goes to court, your report, the police officer's report, and the manager's report will be subpoenaed. Once the judge, prosecuting attorney, and defense attorney read the report, the chance that you will waste any time in court will be minimal.

Example 2. You are called to the scene of an assault where shots have been fired; the scene is unsafe. Once the scene is secured by the police, you are directed into the bedroom, where the patient is lying on the bed in a supine position, arms to the side, legs crossed, with blood about the face and chest. You question your patient about what happened and he responds: "I don't wantyou, I didn't call you, get out." The police interrupt and state that they called EMS to take care of him medically. The patient refuses to cooperate. The police tell you that he was beaten with a baseball bat. You ask him person, place, and time. He answers appropriately. You suggest that the patient undergo a cursory medical. The patient refuses, shouting obscenities at you and your partner.

The police ask your medical opinion of the possibilities. You state that due to the blood about his head and chest, and the violent verbal nature of the patient, the worst-case scenario could possibly be a head injury, chest injury, or lung and/or cardiac contusion. Whatever the case or the possibility, the patient needs to be evaluated at a hospital. You also state to the officer that the possibility of drugs or alcohol is present, which may be the reason for the violent outburst or the assault.

We have a problem here—that the police department really has no cause to forcibly make this person go to the hospital. They also have a responsibility to the patient. However, because of the amount of blood present, the mechanism of injury, and the violent nature of the patient, we have to document this very clearly. Because the patient will not allow us to touch him, our report will consist only of observations and what the police stated.

Now document what occurred.

Ambulance 112 was called to the scene of an assault, advised to stage four blocks away until scene was secured by police department. Staged at the corner of Oak and Pine 300 block. Eight minutes later we were advised by our dispatch that the scene was secure. Approached scene, advised by police on scene that the patient is inside, in the back bedroom. Was assaulted by the neighbor with a baseball bat. Patient refused all treatment and transportation. Advised police that patient should be seen by a physician. Patient alert and oriented, extremely belligerent, and verbally abusive.

Patient found on the bed lying down in supine position, arms at his side and lower extremities crossed. Blood about the face, lacerations about the orbits and mandible; not able to determine the degree of injury because of patient refusal for EMS to touch him. Blood over the chest region, not able to determine extent of injury due to patient's unwillingness to cooperate. Respirations of 22 observed. Pulse or blood pressure unable to attain for reasons stated above. Police advised of possible lung and cardiac contusion, chest injuries, and/or head injuries. Advised police commander that patient should be seen by a physician. Patient refused to sign refusal form, police officer witnessed.

In this situation, even if the patient refuses your treatment/transport, you have an obligation to him. The police is going to have to step in with a protective custody statute or mental health statute. Whichever the case, the police should decide the legal avenue to take. However, this patient must be evaluated by a higher medical authority (i.e., a physician). It is your responsibility to see that this is carried through.

In both scenarios, reference was made to police help. In some situations or in some areas of the country, police are not always on the scene. In some areas police do not want to get involved in the evaluation/refusal process. However, they too are a part of the EMS system as a whole and are also responsible. Do not allow the refusal to be your sole source of patient referral; other avenues for more extensive treatment are available throughout the United States. It is your job to recognize this and act appropriately.

Psychiatric Incidents

Psychiatric patients are hardest to deal with. As emergency care workers we are not trained to communicate with a psychiatric patient. However, these situations do arise and transport/treatment can be refused. In some states the laws allow treatment and transport under implied consent. In some cases the patient may be so violent that physical restraint will have to be used. An on-scene judgment has to be made as to whether such restraint will aggravate the injury. This question should always be in the back of our minds. In either case the points in question will have to be documented.

The problem that we as emergency care givers may face is the situation of a psychiatric patient who has been involved in an accident or who has a medically life-threatening illness. This can present the patient as an extremely violent individual. Because the signs and symptoms are less defined on the psychiatric level, this can put you, as the EMS provider, into a hazardous position.

Physical examinations of psychiatric patients present a most difficult task. Head, neck, and chest exams should be performed with extreme caution regarding your personal safety. Any chest exam involving a female patient should be done by a female health care worker when available.

Hysteria may develop and the examination postponed until the patient is calmed. Suicidal thoughts, destructive behavior, and aggressive behavior must be documented as the incident progresses. Basically, the documentation should specify how the incident progressed, in chronological order.

Whenever restraints are to be used, you must first establish the need for use of the device. Once that need has been made clear to both the EMS staff and the police department, enough support personnel should be on hand to control the patient. Before adequate restraints are applied, have the police department physically search for weapons.

If there is drug involvement, document the type of drugs ingested and proceed accordingly. Actual determination of the cause of the incident is not within the realm of your expertise; however, any information that can be given to the emergency room staff will aid in proper patient care.

In essence we are dealing with two areas: (1) the nonemergent psychiatric patient, and (2) the emergent psychiatric patient. With the nonemergent patient we can take our time gathering information. We can ask particular questions of the patient to document medical problems. If the patient does not want treatment or transport, we have time to investigate other avenues of help.

However, with the emergent psychiatric patient, the situation is more difficult; extreme diplomacy must be taken. This is especially important if the patient is conscious or semiconscious. Consideration of other injuries that are not obvious must be considered, if restraints must be used. If the patient is in such a frame of mind that he or she will listen to reassurance, consider "talking down" the patient.

In either case the best course of action is to create a "relationship" with the patient. The EMS person who has the ability to establish rapport with the patient should be the person who takes care of the patient until you arrive at the hospital.

There are two basic concepts to remember when dealing with this type of patient: (1) find out and document the history and medication of the patient—this will give the medical staff a base to work from; and (2) if restraints are necessary (i.e., to protect the patient and the public), a full assessment of your patient needs to be accomplished prior to emergency room arrival. Pay particular attention to the extremities before and after applying restraint. They may have been placed too tight, limiting the circulation to a particular extremity or all four. Document your assessment with the application of restraints.

Document the entire incident as a progression of events—a chronological timetable, if you will, remembering that every incident is important in accessing an event. Always remember that all patients should be treated with the utmost respect.

Accusation of Incompetence

All who are involved with medicine are aware of the medical–legal atmosphere. However, there is an area of health care that has the responsibility to govern and review the health care process. Within this process of review come questions of negligence—a breech or an omission of an act that could or did have an impact on the well-being of your patient. For ease of discussion and brevity we discuss only the types of cases that may involve the field health care provider. An accusation of incompetent behavior can be handled in a diplomatic fashion if the proper mechanism for handling such a situation is clearly defined. If your service or system does not have such a system, start to generate interest within the system on forming a board for such a purpose.

Over my seventeen years as a health care provider I have seen and have been involved with several cases that involved conflict and/or possible incompetence. In all cases documentation was the key to proof of innocence. A prudent and reasonable EMS provider in each case limited damages due to a well-documented incident. Three that I witnessed went to court. In each case the written report was the pivotal or governing factor as to the outcome of decision.

What we are talking about is a mechanism that holds accountability while controlling medical competence, placing responsibility on the EMS provider. By having such a mechanism in place you are adding credibility to the system as a whole.

Medical control clearly defines the increasing level of who is responsible. Under certain circumstances we are all responsible for our own actions; however, this categorization can be looked at as levels of authority. We can outline these levels into four distinct categories:

1. Supervisor
2. Manager
3. Medical director
4. Board of investigation

The first level is the supervisor, the person who interacts with the field units on a daily basis. This person should be responsible for all the actions of the staff members under him or her. If a question of incompetence arises, it is the supervisor who should investigate the accusation. Verbal accusations can be construed as personal conflicts or personal indifferences. All inquiries should be stated in writing. By recording the differences, the precise level of discrepancy can be addressed. There should be two avenues for grievance: one against the accused and the accused against the originator. In each case and in either direction, the supervisor must look at the facts on hand and make an *objective* decision.

If this level does not satisfy both parties involved, the next step is the manager. He or she has ultimate responsibility for all actions within the service. Again, all generated inquiries should be directed to this person, both the grieving party's documentation regarding the case and the recommendation of the supervisor, together with the reason the recommendation was not acceptable.

The medical director has and holds ultimate responsibility for all emergency providers working within the system. This person should be well versed in the actions, training, and standard procedures of the service. The medical director should provide time to interact and ride with the individual crews in order to observe patient interaction and technical skill level. He or she should also review at random the medical reports that are produced after a call, looking for medical conformity and correct procedural compliance. If the grievance process reaches this level, a formal investigation should take place. Identify areas that either need to be addressed in future training, or disciplinary action incurred on both parties until a just decision can be made. Once this level is reached, all material that has been generated until now should be organized in chronological order and both sides of the story thoroughly investigated by objective parties.

The last level is made up of a board of peers, individuals who interact or have interacted with the parties in question—not friends but people who have worked together in a similar circumstance. The board's membership should be odd-numbered so that when a decision is made, the majority will rule. The peer review board should be made up of all levels of prehospital care providers, an emergency medical technician, a paramedic, an ED nurse (a flight nurse or field nurse would also be appropriate), a physician (other than the medical director), and two laypersons. This board should set up general goals and objectives at which the peer review will look. Areas of discussion may be, but are not limited to, the following: Was there compliance with the local standard of care, taking into consideration the circumstances surrounding the situation? Was the protocol breached, or was the reasoning of the provider in charge appropriate? Was discovery and response done in a timely manner; in other words, was the incident long enough ago to be tainted by time? Was the poor patient outcome a result of the actions that were undertaken? Was degrading of service or negligence involved? The list can go on, depending on the situation and the grievance implied. The board makes the final decision and has the authority to put corrective action in place.

Other Miscellaneous Incidents

Unfortunately, we are living in a world of violence. Acts of aggression in systems comprise a majority of calls. We could elaborate on each category; however, this is beyond the scope of this book. For documentation purposes the following is a list of incidents that require police involvement. The proper authorities should be contacted either by you as a prehospital care provider or the hospital. In some states the responsibility for authority notification lies with both the receiving medical facility and the prehospital care provider, who should be cognizant of the local laws governing such incidents as

Animal bites
Elderly abuse
Battered women
Attempted suicides
Child abuse
Sexual battery
Gunshot wounds
Violent acts of aggression

All such cases should be documented in the same fashion as we documented the psychiatric patient: as a chronological course of events listing all persons involved on the scene, what was said, and all pertinent information. In these situations some states require that special reports be filled out and filed with the proper authorities. In any event, your system and individual service should record such information and keep it on file in the event of future litigation.

Incidents Involving Hazardous Materials

During the past few years hazardous materials awareness has grown phenomenally. New terminology includes *hazardous materials awareness, first* response, specialist, technician, and *Hazwoper,* to name a few. Every industry, place of employment, and emergency response group on one level or another is involved with hazardous materials. The chemicals are too numerous to describe, and some of the literature refers to quantities of material housed within a particular firm or industry, or generally glossed over in groups of classifications.

Our exposure to one or another form of chemical occurs almost on a daily basis. Our bodies usually adjust accordingly. However, if we are in the business to mediate an incident, our exposure may involve a higher concentration than our bodies are able to adjust to. We may be involved with an incident where suit failure has occurred, or repetitive low-dose exposures. Whatever the circumstances, health care providers should take steps to document the exposure.

Exposure functions on two levels: (1) acute, short term, over a short period of time, and (2) chronic, long term, over a long period of time. Both are devastating, depending on the chemical and its concentration.

To protect ourselves from future medical complications, necessary precautions should be taken wherever there are chemicals. Proper respiratory protection should be worn. If the atmosphere promotes skin absorption, the appropriate suit must be donned. As part of the process, an effective decontamination should be part of the procedures. Even if exposure has not taken place, an annual physical should be mandatory to protect all employees involved in any incident.

This introduces us to the first level of medical control: a program that surveys all employees, a medical surveillance program. Such a program creates a baseline of medical data. By establishing the preexisting health of the individual we can be alerted to any problems that may enter the picture. By no means will this save the person from possible problems; what it will do, however, is to create a basis for treatment, medical retirement, or reassignment to another job that may be less stressful and hazardous. Hazardous material incident stabilization is a very demanding task. Not only are we concerned with the medical scope, but we are interested in the mental stress that may be involved.

A qualified physician should be in charge of the medical control program, which includes annual checkups along with a postincident physical as necessary. But what happens on the scene of a HAZ-MAT situation? What can we do as the providers in the field?

The run report on a hazardous materials incident requires a unique set of information. I suggest a run report that includes the following: First establish a general standard operating procedure (SOP) as to how a hazardous materials incident will be answered—not from a tactical standpoint but from a medical one. This SOP should provide guidance for the medical surveillance program (how to enter it, who to contact, what paperwork needs to be completed) as well as procedures for preincident and postincident. It should also outline any medical procedures that will take place once an exposure has occurred.

The medical surveillance SOP should be incorporated with your department's standard approach for handling annual physicals and on-the-job injury. This area will be for the most part regional in nature and will not be discussed on a specific level here.

Pre- and postincident management is something we can do as prehospital providers. We are called to an incident. Depending on our job description, we will be more or less involved with a HAZ-MAT operation. To protect the persons who must enter the location involved, baseline care must be provided.

Blood pressure, pulse, respirations (including auscultation), blood samples, and an electrocardiogram (EKG) are within the capability of all prehospital providers. Hydration is yet another consideration. Once the persons involved are decontaminated, another set of vitals and blood work can be developed, all being documented for later reference.

Following is an example of a pre- and postincident report that can be used as a documentation tool. (See Figure 3-1.) I have listed general information. The first is time in, time out, which establishes a time frame of exposure—important if suit or equipment failure has taken place. Then, how long the person was in the decontamination process, and whether this was exposure or actual material contact. An addition that was not placed on the health or HAZ-MAT team document, because it falls more in line with the safety officer's documentation rather than the medical sector's, is the amount of air respired if a self-contained breathing apparatus was used. This respiratory information or documentation will help the medical staff at the hospital to determine an approximate inhaled chemical potential. I have listed eight procedures that should be performed prior to entrance into a Haz-Mat incident. Four of these should be performed upon completion of decontamination at intervals of 1 and 5 minutes:

Blood pressure
Respirations
Pulse rate
Pulse oximetry

Other considerations are:

EKG (12 lead if available)
Lung sounds
Hydration
Blood drawn for testing

Initially we took blood, red top, purple top, blue top, green top (your local lab may have different color designations for the various tests), full blood chemistry, including liver function, blood forming tests, hematocrit, hemoglobin, and heavy metals. These tests should be given to all persons involved in the incident. (See Figures 3-2 and 3-3.) If an actual exposure occurs, the rest of the form can be filled out. As you can see, it establishes a medical report for the hospital utilizing the systems approach in a checkoff list fashion. The end of the report includes areas for specific medical interaction and drug antidotes that may be used at the scene or during transport.

As with all checkoff reports, a comment section is included. Items to document:

Type of chemical
Equipment used for personal protection
Treatment initiated
Decontamination
Possible concentration
List of previous exposure
Temperature and humidity
Response to treatment
Transportation decontamination

DATE ________, INCIDENT # ________, UNIT ________

INCIDENT ADDRESS ________

MATERIAL: CHEMICAL NAME ________

U.N.I.D. # ________, TRADE/COMMON NAME ________

PRIMARY ENTRY TEAM

Patient's Name ☐ Age: ☐ Sex ☐ Male ☐ Female ☐ Wt. in kg

Time In: ☐ Time Out: ☐ Decon Time: ☐

Exposure ☐ Yes ☐ No

	INIT	1 MIN	5 MIN
Blood Prussure	/	/	/
Pulse Rate			
Respirations			
Pulse Oximetry			

EKG ________
Hydrate ________
Lung Sounds ________
Blood Drawn R☐ P☐ B☐ G☐

PRIMARY ENTRY TEAM

Patient's Name ☐ Age: ☐ Sex ☐ Male ☐ Female ☐ Wt. in kg

Time In: ☐ Time Out: ☐ Decon Time: ☐

Exposure ☐ Yes ☐ No

	INIT	1 MIN	5 MIN
Blood Prussure	/	/	/
Pulse Rate			
Respirations			
Pulse Oximetry			

EKG ________
Hydrate ________
Lung Sounds ________
Blood Drawn R☐ P☐ B☐ G☐

BACK-UP ENTRY TEAM

Patient's Name ☐ Age: ☐ Sex ☐ Male ☐ Female ☐ Wt. in kg

Time In: ☐ Time Out: ☐ Decon Time: ☐

Exposure ☐ Yes ☐ No

	INIT	1 MIN	5 MIN
Blood Prussure	/	/	/
Pulse Rate			
Respirations			
Pulse Oximetry			

EKG ________
Hydrate ________
Lung Sounds ________
Blood Drawn R☐ P☐ B☐ G☐

BACK-UP ENTRY TEAM

Patient's Name ☐ Age: ☐ Sex ☐ Male ☐ Female ☐ Wt. in kg

Time In: ☐ Time Out: ☐ Decon Time: ☐

Exposure ☐ Yes ☐ No

	INIT	1 MIN	5 MIN
Blood Prussure	/	/	/
Pulse Rate			
Respirations			
Pulse Oximetry			

EKG ________
Hydrate ________
Lung Sounds ________
Blood Drawn R☐ P☐ B☐ G☐

FIGURE 3-1 *Preincident form.*

PRIMARY ENTRY TEAM

Patient's Name ______ Age: ☐ Sex ☐ Male ☐ Female ______ Wt. in kg

Time In: ☐ Time Out: ☐ Decon Time: ☐

Exposure ☐ Yes ☐ No

	INIT	1 MIN	5 MIN
Blood Prussure	/	/	/
Pulse Rate			
Respirations			
Pulse Oximetry			

EKG ______
Hydrate ______
Lung Sounds ______
Blood Drawn R☐ P☐ B☐ G☐

Notes: ______

Chief Complaint: " ______ "

P.I: ______

(Location, Quality, Intensity, Quantity, Cronology, Setting, Scenario of First Symptoms, Aggravation and Alleviation, Associated Complaints, Attempts to Modify)

P.M.I:

General state of health ______

Past illnesses: ☐ Heart Disease ☐ Ulcers ☐ Emphysema ☐ Hypertension ☐ Asthma ☐ Cancer ☐ Diabetes ☐ Other } ______

Hospitalizations (include psychiatric illnesses): ______

Surgery: ______

Allergies: ______ Include environmental, ingestible or drug related!

Immunizations: ______

Substance Abuse (include alcohol, cigarettes, and street drugs: ______

Medications (include over the counter meds): ______

Mental: ☐ Conscious ☐ Alert ☐ Unconscious ☐ Oriented { Person ☐ Place ☐ Time ☐

Status: ☐ Restless ☐ Co-operative ☐ Combative ☐ Other ______

Skin: ☐ Warm ☐ Cool ☐ Mottled ☐ Diaphoretic ☐ Flushed ☐ Pink ☐ Dry ☐ Clammy ☐ Cyanotic ☐ Jaundice ☐ Pallor ☐ Other ______

Pupils: ☐ PEARL ☐ Other ______ **Size:** OD ☐ OS ☐ **Vis. Acuity:** OD ☐/ OS ☐/

Skull: ______ (Describe)

ENT: ☐ Draining ☐ Difficulty swallowing ☐ Post Nasal ☐ Other ______

Face: ______ (Describe)

FIGURE 3-2 *Postincident form if exposed.*

Neck: ☐ Supple ☐ Engorged Veins ☐ Nuchal Rigidity ☐ Other ____________

Chest: Heart Sounds: ☐ S1 ☐ S2 ☐ S3 ☐ Muffled ☐ Other ____________

Lungs: ☐ Clear ☐ Rales ☐ Rhonchi ☐ Other

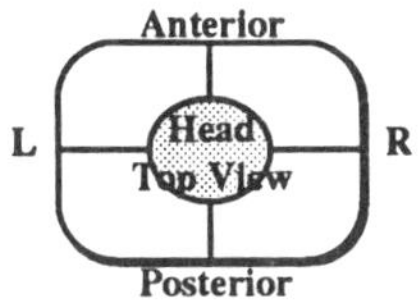

Resp: ☐ Shallow ☐ Labored ☐ Retraction ______ ☐ Deep ☐ SOB ☐ Injury ______ ☐ Slow ☐ Effortless ☐ Rapid ☐ Kussmaul ☐ Rate

Abdomen: ☐ Soft ☐ Rebound ☐ Distended ☐ Guarding ☐ Rigid ☐ Nausea ☐ Swollen ☐ Emesis ____________

UL	UR
LL	LR

√ Bowel Sounds

G.U: ☐ Burning ☐ Urgency ☐ Color ______ ☐ Frequency ☐ Hematuria ☐ Other ______

GYN: (State "Male" if so) ☐ Bleeding Discharge ______ ☐ LMP ______ ☐ Para ______ ☐ Gravida ______ ☐ Ab ______

Spine: ____________ (Describe)

Extremity:

Injury: ____________ Pulses: ______

☐ Warm ☐ Cyanotic ☐ Pink ☐ Mottled ☐ Cool ☐ Edema ______ ☐ Color ______

☐ Weakness Handgrasp ☐ Movement Dorsiflexion

Left Arm	Rt. Arm	Left Leg	Rt. Leg

Vital Signs:

Time						
Sys/Dia	/	/	/	/	/	/
Pulse						
Resp.						
Temp.						

Cardiac Monitor

EKG

		Amt	Time	Amt	Time	Amt	Time	Amt	Time	Amt	Time
Respiratory	Epinephrine										
	Alupent Nebulizer										
	Alupent Inhaler										
	Brethine										
Cyanide	Amyl Nitrite Pearls										
	Sodium Nitrite										
	Sodium Thiosulfate										
Unconscious	Thiamine										
	$D_{50}W$										
Eye	Ponticane Hypochloride										
	Sodium Chloride										
Organic Phosphate	Atropine										
	2 PAM Chloride										
	Valium										
Nitrites/Nitrates	Methylene Blue										
Fluoride Salts	Calcium Gluconate										

(Comments) ____________

____________ Signature ______ Date

FIGURE 3-2 *continued*

Clinical Narrative

Date:

Location:

Clinical:

FIGURE 3-3 *Comments narrative to exposure form.*

4

Assessment Report Categories

The next three chapters and the appendix are your reference sections. With what we learned in the first three chapters, we can use the information lists as possible written objectives. As we discussed in Chapter 2, the considerations that one must observe, remember, and document are lengthy. However, I have put together lists that will aid you in writing a report.

There are three different approaches. First we take the most common one, patient assessment, and apply it to report writing: the head-to-toe survey. Next we take the head-to-toe survey and modify it with the nursing aspect of evaluation, keeping in mind rapid scene evaluation: the body systems approach. Finally, we look at it from the angle of the type incident: the call incident approach.

It is set up so that you can include and combine a variety of approaches. This is acceptable. However, because each section and subsection of each approach was designed to stand alone, be aware of redundancy. Many students and seasoned rescuers find that using the call incident approach in association with the head-to-toe method generates the type of report they like. Flight medics and nurses seem to use the systems-approach highlighted areas from the call incident section. It does not matter how you utilize the reference text; again, it was designed for the field rescuer/EMS provider and can be used in a variety of ways according to individual needs, each correct in its use and function.

HEAD-TO-TOE APPROACH

In this section we utilize the secondary head-to-toe approach as the avenue to report writing. The head-to-toe survey is an organized approach to evaluate a patient; therefore, it is logical to use the same procedure to write what we find.

I have organized this approach into six areas. The first five deal with considerations other than the assessment itself. It places in order some basic and some advanced considerations. Subjective and objective questions are sometimes placed together, to jog your memory to incorporate additional informative facts in the document.

General Overview

Observation: Observe the obvious bleeding, swelling, deformity, discharge, discoloration, tenderness, respirational patterns, skin color, and temperature.

History/Chief Complaint: What event(s) precipitated the problem for which you were called—both past events and recent events?

Special Considerations: Is the patient in an environment that can be or is dangerous, such as weather exposure, mechanism of injury, dangerous scene, or potential of becoming very dangerous?

Head to Toe: Starting with the head and working toward the feet, *look* by inspection, *listen* by auscultation, and *feel* by palpation and percussion to gain the needed information.

Observations

- Observe the patient continuously, noting:

Bleeding	Swelling
Deformity	Discoloration
Respirations	Discharge
Skin color	Temperature

- Is the patient trying to tell you something?
- Has your patient's level of consciousness remained the same?
- Can the patient tell you what happened?
- Does the patient remember what happened?
- Do any of the bystanders have any information?

History/Chief Complaint

- Relevant past history
- Smoking: quantity
- Has a similar event happened before; if so, under what circumstances?
- Relevant recent history
- Recent contact with a hazardous atmosphere.
- How long has this particular problem been present?
- Different life-style or behavioral patterns
- Incident with or without activity
- Hypotension/hypertension
- Allergies
- Medical ID tag present (around neck, wrist, or wallet)
- Activity before EMS arrival
- Approximate time problem started

- Acute or chronic condition
- Was the event abrupt or gradual?

Special Considerations

- Is the scene safe for the rescuer and the patient?
- Does the patient need rapid removal from the immediate scene?
- Child abuse
- Scene dangerous or becoming dangerous to the patient and/or rescue workers?
- Does the patient need rapid transport?
- Mechanism of injury present
- Elderly abuse
- Surrounding environment: Medications, alcohol, narcotics, contraband
- Weather exposure harmful?

Head to Toe

VITAL SIGNS

Pulse	• Rate	• Rhythm	• Quality
Respirations	• Rate	• Quantity	• Quality
Blood pressure	• Hyper/hypotension		• Equal bilaterally
	• Pulse pressure		• Orthostatic
Skin color/ temperature	**Color**	**Temp.**	**Condition**
	• Cyanosis	• Warm/dry	• Mottling
	• Redness	• Warm/wet	• Turgor
	• Jaundice	• Hot/wet	
		• Hot/dry	
		• Cool/wet	
		• Cool/dry	
Eyes	• Pupils reactive to light, equal; size		
	• Moist/dry, round/symmetrical pupils		
	• Sclera color: yellow, bloodshot		
Ability to move	• Move to command	• Reaction to pain	
	• Upper extremities	• Lower extremities	
Level of consciousness	• Alert and oriented to person, place, and time		
	• Appropriate/inappropriate behavior		
	• Confused, unintelligible sounds		
	• Spontaneous eye opening		
	• Easily aroused, obeys commands		

HEAD

Observations: Deformity, discoloration, swelling, facial muscle tone, discharge from the nose and/or ears, petechiae, mental status, pain either local or general, bleeding.

Eyes	• Ecchymosis (raccoon eyes)	• Equal and reactive
	• Cataracts/glaucoma	• Contacts

Pupils	• Pinpoint • Symmetric	• Midsize	• Dilated
Sclera	• Petechiae	• Jaundiced	• Red
Conjunctiva	• Pale	• Inflamed	• Lack of tears
Ears	• Ecchymosis (Battle's sign)		• Discharge
Nose	• Discoloration • Drainage of fluid • Singed nasal hairs	• Deformity	• Flaring of the nares
Mouth	• Cyanosis of the mucosa • Furrowed tongue	• Lack of saliva	• Singed lips • Burned mouth • Alcohol/acetone

NECK

Observations: Deformity, discoloration, swelling, subcutaneous emphysema, cyanosis, petechiae, bleeding.

- Tracheal tugging
- Nuchal rigidity
- Subcutaneous emphysema
- Distended neck veins
- Tracheal deviation

CHEST

Observations: Deformity, discoloration, swelling, subcutanous emphysema, cyanosis, petechiae, bleeding.

- Rate
- Intercostal retractions
- Auscultation of the lungs: rales, rhonchi stridor, wheezing, snoring
- Kussmauls (hypopenea-tachypenea)
- Cheyne-Stokes (increase-decrease-apnea)
- Symmetrical movements
- Accessory muscle retractions
- Apnea
- Volume
- Effort: quality, quantity
- Barrel chest
- Pain
  - Location
  - Duration
  - Radiation
  - Nature of pain
  - Pressure
  - Sharp Mild
  - Dull Sudden
  - Slow onset
- Open wounds
- Paradoxical
- Tach/bradypnea
- Respiratory patterns
- Coughing: mucus productive/ nonproductive:
  - Thick: yellow, green
  - Foamy: pink/red, white, clear/yellow
- Sternal retractions
- Crepitus
- Flail segment
- Symmetry equal
- Orthopnea

UPPER EXTREMITIES

Observations: Deformity, discoloration, swelling, cyanosis, petechiae, bleeding.

- Pain
- Distal pulses
- Paralysis
- Posturing
- Equal grip strength
- Numbness
- Equal pulses
- Paresthesia
- Capillary refill
- Point tenderness
- Skin temperature
- Skin color
- Skin turgor

ABDOMEN

Observations: Deformity, discoloration, swelling, muscle tone, pain, cyanosis, petechiae, bleeding.

- Point tenderness
- Abrasions
- Rigidity
- Pain upon palpation
- Skin color
- Masses noted
- Open wounds
- Guarding
- Ecchymosis

PELVIS

Observations: Deformity, discoloration, swelling, muscle tone, pain, cyanosis, petechiae, bleeding.

- Point tenderness
- Abrasions
- Bleeding: rectal/vaginal
- Ecchymosis
- Pain upon palpation
- Skin color
- Open wounds
- Guarding
- Masses noted

LOWER EXTREMITIES

Observations: Deformity, discoloration, swelling, cyanosis, petechiae, bleeding.

- Pain
- Distal pulses
- Paralysis
- Posturing
- Rotation: internal/external
- Numbness
- Equal pulses
- Paresthesia
- Capillary refill
- Point tenderness
- Skin temperature
- Skin color
- Skin turgor
- Shortening

BODY SYSTEMS APPROACH

In this section each body system is subdivided into the following areas:

History
Pulse
Blood pressure
Respiration
Skin color/temperature
Pupils
Level of consciousness
Ability to move
Reaction to pain

History: Any information that accurately builds an account of the sick or injured person. The history of a patient is very important to the physician, the hospital, and the rescue worker. As health care providers we need to record as much information as possible that contributes to the basic understanding of recent past events, past medical events, and any event that might have precipitated the emergency call.

Pulse: When evaluating the pulse, the rescue worker must choose the most appropriate pulse point for the situation. There are eight basic pulse points that can be used: apical, carotid, brachial, radial, femoral, popliteal, pedial, lateral tibial. Capillary refill is perhaps the best indicator of perfusion to the vital organs. If we see good capillary refill, we can assume that the organs are also being well perfused.

Blood Pressure: Placement and appropriate cuff size are the two parameters that are dealt with when taking a blood pressure. These parameters must always be in the back of your mind when assessing a patient. In addition to the rapid increase and decrease of both the systolic and diasytolic pressures, a decreasing pulse pressure should also be noted in both arms. Positional or orthostatic blood pressures should also be assessed. Palpating a blood pressure is sometimes necessary. Remember that when this procedure is done, the value obtained is 3 to 8 mmHg lower than the auscultated method. Blood pressure taken from the popliteal is also possible, but again there can be a decrease of 8 to 10 mmHg.

Respiration: This area is sometimes overlooked. One must recall how the lung is constructed. There are two lung fields, the right lung being larger and heavier than the left. Each lung has an apex and a base. The apex forms a tapering cone at the top, and the base forms a broad concave surface at the bottom. As the chest muscles constrict, the chest is brought up and out, decreasing the atmospheric pressure within the lung space; thus air rushes in, enabling us to breathe. Remember when auscultating the lungs check the apex and the bases, both anteriorly and posteriorly. Depth of breath, equality of expansion, and volume inhaled should be noted. Pulse oximerty—the new "vital sign"—is related to respiration. These devices measure the percent saturation of oxygen in the blood. Although these devices have their drawbacks, percentages above 94%, together with good observable respiratory drive, establish a good baseline for the respiratory status of the patient.

Skin color/Temperature: Initial color should always be noted along with the temperature of the skin. This sign describes the adequacy of perfusion, *not* oxygenation. Although they are closely related, good oxygenation does not always mean good perfusion. Temperature of the skin can also give the direction of the patient's condition.

Pupils: The pupillary response has been reported as the window to the brain. Although in some cases this might be true, it is not always the case. A continuous evaluation of the pupils' reaction to light and the placement within the orbit should be documented. The normal size of the adult pupil is approximately 2 to 3 mm, bilaterally symmetric, unless there is an underlying disease, trauma, or drugs. Note whether they are bilaterally dilated, constricted, pinpoint, fixed, fully dilated, or midpoint.

Level of Consciousness: Terms such as *lethargic, stupor,* and *comatose* should not be used to describe the patient in the prehospital setting. Such terms lend themselves to a high degree of misunderstanding between the rescuer and the receiving physician. A description of the neurologically impaired patient is needed. The description of the activity must be evaluated and documented with terms such as "alert, oriented to person, time, and place"; "confused, uses inappropriate words, obeys commands, spontaneous eye movement" better describes the level of consciousness. Remember that the abbreviation LOC does not stand for "loss of consciousness" but for "level of consciousness."

Ability to Move: The ability to move shows the rescuer the patient's ability to understand a command associated with a motor response. The postural attitude of the patient displays the possible injury level that the cerebral cortex might have sustained. *Decerebrate* posturing displays the possibility of upper brainstem damage; the legs are extended with the feet flexed, and the arms are extended with the hands clinched and pulled inward. The head is erect and the jaw clenched. *Decorticate* posturing displays possible injury to the brain's cortex. This type of posturing is seen more in children than in adults. It is described as an extension of the legs with the feet rotated inward and extended. The arms are flexed. *Flaccid* posturing indicates a spinal cord injury.

Reaction to Pain: This tests the patient's ability to react to a stimulus in either an appropriate or an inappropriate manner. Does the patient react to local pain, withdraw from the pain, or move toward the pain stimulus? Is there movement at all with pain stimulus?

In addition to the history, which is subjective, the following objective information should be collected. In each subcategory: look by inspection, listen by auscultation, and feel by palpation to gain the needed information. Any mechanism of injury must be investigated further. Strenuous activity or lack of activity should be reported.

The chief complaint is the patient's description of the problem (symptoms) and can be categorized in the following general areas:

1. Intensity
2. Aggravation
3. Quality
4. Location
5. Alleviation
6. Quantity
7. Environment
8. History
9. Duration

The body systems approach to report writing is organized into the following categories:

1. Cardiovascular system
2. Respiratory system
3. Central nervous system
4. Musculoskeletal system
5. Reproductive system
6. General medical

1. The Cardiovascular System

History:

- Relevant distant history
- Smoking: quantity
- Has a similar event happened before; if so, under what circumstances?
- Acute or chronic?
- Gradual or abrupt?
- Hypotension
- Hypertension
- Activity before EMS arrival
- Incident with or without activity
- Recent history
- Recent contact with hazardous atmosphere
- How long has the patient had this particular complaint?
- Medications and dose/allergies
- How was patient found?
- Position patient found

Pulse:

- Pulse, rate, rhythm quality
- Distended neck veins
- Degree of capillary refill
- Pedal edema

Blood pressure:	• Orthostatic blood pressure	• Pulse pressure • Equal pressure in both arms
Respiratory:	• Respiratory effort: quantity, quality • Equal bilaterally • Retraction of intercostal muscles • Coughing: sputum color Thick: yellow/green Foamy: pink/red White: clear/yellow • Auscultation of the lungs Rales Rhonchi Wheezing Stridor Snoring (location wet/dry—rate/volume) • Nausea and vomiting • Kussmauls (hyperpnea–tachypnea) • Pulse oximerty	• Tracheal tugging • Nasal flaring • Diaphragmatic breathing • Abdominal muscle use • Pain, nature of: Pressure (squeezing) Sharp Mild/dull Sudden/slow onset Radiation of pain Location of pain Duration of pain Distant lung sounds • Cheyne–Stokes (increase–apnea–increase)
Skin color and temperature:	• Cyanosis • Redness • Yellow • Mottling • Turgor • Diaphoresis: extreme, mild, moderate.	• Warm/dry • Warm/wet • Cool/dry • Cool/wet • Hot/dry • Hot/wet
Pupils:	• Equal and reactive to light • Glaucoma • Pupils: pinpoint, midsize • Dilated, symmetric, round • Conjunctiva: pale, inflamed, red, lack of tears	• Cataracts • Contacts • Sclera: petechiae jaundiced, bloodshot
Level of consciousness:	• Easily aroused • Alert and oriented to person, place, and time • Appropriate words • Inappropriate behavior	• Confused • Obeys commands • Spontaneous eye opening
Ability to move:	• Seizure activity: postictal, grand mal, focal	• Flexation/extension • Grip strength • Pain upon movement

Trauma-related cases:

- Muffled heart sounds
- Discolored region
- Chest region cyanotic
- Battle's sign
- Swollen tongue
- Deformity
- Bloodshot scalera
- Raccoon eyes
- Flail chest section
- Engorged neck veins

2. The Respiratory System

History:

- Relevant distant history
- Smoking: quantity
- Has a similar event happened before; if so, under what circumstances?
- Acute or chronic?
- Gradual or abrupt?
- Asthma
- Emphysema
- COPD
- Time distress started
- Incident with or without activity
- Activity before EMS arrival
- Recent history
- Recent contact with hazardous atmosphere
- How long has the patient had this particular complaint?
- Medications and dose/allergies
- How was patient found?
- Position patient found

Pulse:

- Pulse, rate, rhythm quality
- Distended neck veins
- Degree of capillary refill
- Pedal edema

Blood pressure:

- Orthostatic blood pressure
- Pulse pressure
- Equal pressure in both arms

Respiratory:

- Respiratory effort: quantity, quality
- Equal bilaterally
- Retraction of intercostal muscles
- Coughing: sputum color
  Thick: yellow/green
  Foamy: pink/red
  White: clear/yellow
- Auscultation of the lungs
  Rales Rhonchi
  Wheezing Stridor
  Snoring
  (location wet/dry—rate/volume)
- Nausea and vomiting
- Kussmauls (hyperpnea–tachypnea)
- Tracheal tugging
- Nasal flaring
- Diaphragmatic breathing
- Abdominal muscle use
- Pain, nature of:
  Pressure (squeezing)
  Sharp
  Mild/dull
  Sudden/slow onset
  Radiation of pain
  Location of pain
  Duration of pain
  Distant lung sounds
- Cheyne–Stokes (increase–apnea–increase)
- Pain associated with inspiration/expiration

	• Pulse oximerty • Barrel chest • Volume of breath • Biot's (apnea–hyperpnea)	
Skin color and temperature:	• Cyanosis • Redness • Yellow • Mottling • Turgor • Diaphoresis: extreme, mild, moderate	• Warm/dry • Warm/wet • Cool/dry • Cool/wet • Hot/dry • Hot/wet
Pupils:	• Equal and reactive to light • Glaucoma • Pupils: pinpoint, midsize • Dilated, symmetric, round • Conjunctiva: pale, inflamed, red, lack of tears	• Cataracts • Contacts • Sclera: petechiae jaundiced, bloodshot
Level of consciousness:	• Easily aroused • Alert and oriented to person, place, and time • Appropriate words • Inappropriate behavior	• Confused • Obeys commands • Spontaneous eye opening
Ability to move:	• Seizure activity: postictal, grand mal, focal	• Flexation/extension • Grip strength • Pain upon movement
Trauma-related cases:	• Subcutanous emphysema • Discolored region • Chest region cyanotic • Battle's sign • Swollen tongue • Distant lung sounds • Muffled heart sounds • Mechanism of injury	• Deformity • Tracheal deviation • Raccoon eyes • Flail chest section • Engorged neck veins • Jugular distension • Singed lips, nares, and mouth

3. The Central Nervous System

History:	• Relevant distant history • Syncopal episode • Has a similar event happened before; if so, under what circumstances?	• Recent history • Recent contact with hazardous atmosphere • How long has the patient had this particular complaint?

- Accident type:
  Auto accident: mph of the vehicles involved, rollover, head-on, side, rear, etc.
- Fall, assault
- Activity before EMS arrival
- Incident with or without activity
- Medications and dose/allergies
- How was patient found?
- Position patient found

Pulse:

- Pulse, rate, rhythm quality
- Distended neck veins
- Degree of capillary refill
- Pedal edema

Blood pressure:

- Orthostatic blood pressure
- Pulse pressure
- Equal pressure in both arms

Respiratory:

- Respiratory effort: quantity, quality
- Equal bilaterally
- Retraction of intercostal muscles
- Distant lung sounds
- Respiratory status with relationship to level of sensorium
- Auscultation of the lungs
  Rales Rhonchi
  Wheezing Stridor
  Snoring
  (location wet/dry—rate/volume)
- Nausea and vomiting
- Kussmauls (hyperpnea–tachypnea)
- Pulse oximerty
- Barrel chest
- Volume of breath
- Biot's (apnea–hyperpnea)
- Tracheal tugging
- Nasal flaring
- Diaphragmatic breathing
- Abdominal muscle use
- Pain, nature of:
  Pressure (squeezing)
  Sharp
  Mild/dull
  Sudden/slow onset
  Radiation of pain
  Location of pain
  Duration of pain
  Distant lung sounds
- Cheyne–Stokes (increase–apnea–increase)
- Pain associated with inspiration/expiration

Skin color and temperature:

- Cyanosis
- Redness
- Yellow
- Mottling
- Turgor
- Diaphoresis: extreme, mild, moderate
- Warm/dry
- Warm/wet
- Cool/dry
- Cool/wet
- Hot/dry
- Hot/wet

Pupils:

- Equal and reactive to light
- Cataracts
- Contacts

- Glaucoma
- Pupils: pinpoint, midsize
- Dilated, symmetric, round
- Conjunctiva: pale, inflamed, red, lack of tears
- Sclera: petechiae jaundiced, bloodshot

Level of consciousness:

- Easily aroused
- Alert and oriented to person, place, and time
- Appropriate words
- Inappropriate behavior
- Confused
- Obeys commands
- Spontaneous eye opening
- Level of sensation

Ability to move:

- Seizure activity: postictal, grand mal, focal
- Ability to discriminate sharp/dull and sensation
- Flexation/extension
- Grip strength
- Pain upon movement

Trauma-related cases:

- Subcutanous emphysema
- Discolored region
- Chest region cyanotic
- Battle's sign
- Swollen tongue
- Distant lung sounds
- Muffled heart sounds
- Mechanism of injury
- Extreme pain
- Ability to move above and below injury site
- Posturing: decorticate/decerebrate
- Deformity
- Tracheal deviation
- Raccoon eyes
- Flail chest section
- Engorged neck veins
- Jugular distension
- Singed lips, nares, and mouth
- Muscle tone
- Pain sharp, dull, burning

4. The Musculoskeletal System

History:

- Relevant distant history
- Syncopal episode
- Has a similar event happened before; if so, under what circumstances?
- Accident type:
  Auto accident: mph of the vehicles involved, rollover, head-on, side, rear, etc.
- Fall, distance
- Activity before EMS arrival
- Incident with or without activity
- Assault
- Recent history
- Recent contact with hazardous atmosphere
- How long has the patient had this particular complaint?
- Medications and dose/allergies
- How was patient found?
- Position patient found

Pulse:

- Pulse, rate, rhythm quality
- Distended neck veins
- Laceration
- Contusions
- Avulsion
- Distal pulse
- Degree of capillary refill
- Pedal edema
- Abrasions
- Puncture wound
- Hematoma
- Penetrating injury

Blood pressure:

- Orthostatic blood pressure
- Pulse pressure
- Equal pressure in both arms

Respiratory:

- Respiratory effort: quantity, quality
- Equal bilaterally
- Retraction of intercostal muscles
- Distant lung sounds
- Respiratory status with relationship to level of sensorium
- Auscultation of the lungs
  - Rales Rhonchi
  - Wheezing Stridor
  - Snoring
  - (location wet/dry—rate/volume)
- Nausea and vomiting
- Kussmauls (hyperpnea–tachypnea)
- Pulse oximerty
- Barrel chest
- Volume of breath
- Tracheal tugging
- Nasal flaring
- Diaphragmatic breathing
- Abdominal muscle use
- Pain, nature of:
  - Pressure (squeezing)
  - Sharp
  - Mild/dull
  - Sudden/slow onset
  - Radiation of pain
  - Location of pain
  - Duration of pain
  - Distant lung sounds
- Cheyne–Stokes (increase–apnea–increase)
- Pain associated with inspiration/expiration

Skin color and temperature:

- Cyanosis
- Redness
- Yellow
- Mottling
- Turgor
- Diaphoresis: extreme, mild, moderate
- Warm/dry
- Warm/wet
- Cool/dry
- Cool/wet
- Hot/dry
- Hot/wet

Pupils:

- Equal and reactive to light
- Glaucoma
- Pupils: pinpoint, midsize
- Dilated, symmetric, round
- Conjunctiva: pale, inflamed, red, lack of tears
- Cataracts
- Contacts
- Sclera: petcchiae jaundiced, bloodshot

Level of consciousness:

- Easily aroused
- Alert and oriented to person, place, and time
- Appropriate words
- Inappropriate behavior
- Confused
- Obeys commands
- Spontaneous eye opening
- Level of sensation

Ability to move:

- Seizure activity: post-ictal, grand mal, focal
- Ability to discriminate sharp/dull and sensation
- Flexation/extension
- Grip strength
- Pain upon movement

Trauma-related cases:

- Subcutanous emphysema
- Discolored region
- Chest region cyanotic
- Battle's sign
- Swollen tongue
- Distant lung sounds
- Muffled heart sounds
- Mechanism of injury
- Extreme pain
- Ability to move above and below injury site
- Posturing: decorticate/decerebrate
- Deformity
- Tracheal deviation
- Raccoon eyes
- Flail chest section
- Engorged neck veins
- Jugular distension
- Singed lips, nares, and mouth
- Muscle tone
- Pain sharp, dull, burning
- Percent burn

5. The Reproductive System

History:

- Relevant distant history
- Smoking: quantity
- Prenatal care/education
- Month of conception: due date
- Hypotension
- Hypertension
- Any vaginal discharge: clear/bloody/clots
- Duration of contractions
- Urinary tract infection
- Amniotic merconium
- Normal/abnormal menstrual cycle
- Feeling of a bowel movement
- Has a similar event happened before; if so, under what circumstances?
- Recent history
- Length of present pregnancy
- Number of pregnancies Live birth, abortions/miscarriages, abnormal events:
  Eclampsia
  Toxemia
  Placenta previa
  Placenta abrupto
- Last menstrual cycle
- Syncopal episode
- Polyuria
- Pedal edema
- Recent contact with hazardous atmosphere
- How long has the patient had this particular complaint?

- Activity before EMS arrival
- Incident with or without activity
- How was patient found?
- Medications and dose/allergies
- Position patient found

Pulse:

- Pulse, rate, rhythm quality
- Distended neck veins
- Hemorrhage
- Degree of capillary refill
- Pedal edema

Blood pressure:

- Orthostatic blood pressure
- Pulse pressure
- Equal pressure in both arms

Respiratory:

- Respiratory effort: quantity, quality
- Equal bilaterally
- Retraction of intercostal muscles
- Coughing: sputum color
  - Thick: yellow/green
  - Foamy: pink/red
  - White: clear/yellow
- Auscultation of the lungs
  - Rales Rhonchi
  - Wheezing Stridor
  - Snoring
  - (location wet/dry—rate/volume)
- Pulse oximetry
- Nausea and vomiting
- Nasal flaring
- Diaphragmatic breathing
- Abdominal muscle use
- Pain, nature of:
  - Pressure (squeezing)
  - Sharp
  - Mild/dull
  - Sudden/slow onset
  - Radiation of pain
  - Location of pain
  - Duration of pain
  - Distant lung sounds

Skin color and Temperature:

- Cyanosis
- Redness
- Yellow
- Mottling
- Turgor
- Diaphoresis: extreme, mild, moderate
- Warm/dry
- Warm/wet
- Cool/dry
- Cool/wet
- Hot/dry
- Hot/wet

Pupils:

- Equal and reactive to light
- Glaucoma
- Pupils: pinpoint, midsize
- Dilated, symmetric, round
- Conjunctiva: pale, inflamed, red, lack of tears
- Cataracts
- Contacts
- Sclera: petechiae jaundiced, bloodshot

Level of consciousness:

- Easily aroused
- Alert and oriented to person, place, and time
- Appropriate words
- Inappropriate behavior
- Confused
- Obeys commands
- Spontaneous eye opening

Ability to move:

- Seizure activity: post-ictal, grand mal, focal
- Flexation/extension
- Grip strength
- Pain upon movement

Trauma-related cases:

- Muffled heart sounds
- Discolored region
- Chest region cyanotic
- Battle's sign
- Swollen tongue
- Fetal heart tones
- Deformity
- Bloodshot scalera
- Raccoon eyes
- Flail chest section
- Engorged neck veins

6. General Medical

History:

- Relevant distant history
- Smoking: quantity
- Has a similar event happened before; if so, under what circumstances?
- Acute or chronic?
- Gradual or abrupt?
- Asthma
- Emphysema
- COPD
- Time distress started
- Incident with or without activity
- Fall: distance
- Activity before EMS arrival
- Chest pain
- Recent history
- Recent contact with hazardous atmosphere
- How long has the patient had this particular complaint?
- Medications and dose/allergies
- How was patient found?
- Position patient found
- Accident type
- Syncopal episode

Pulse:

- Pulse, rate, rhythm quality
- Distended neck veins
- Laceration
- Contusions
- Avulsion
- Distal pulse
- Degree of capillary refill
- Hematoma
- Abrasions
- Puncture wound
- Pulse pressure
- Penetrating injury

Blood pressure:

- Orthostatic blood pressure
- Pulse pressure
- Equal pressure in both arms

Respiratory:

- Respiratory effort: quantity, quality
- Equal bilaterally
- Retraction of intercostal muscles
- Tracheal tugging
- Nasal flaring
- Diaphragmatic breathing
- Abdominal muscle use

- Distant lung sounds
- Respiratory status with relationship to level of sensorium
- Auscultation of the lungs
  - Rales
  - Rhonchi
  - Wheezing
  - Stridor
  - Snoring
  - (location wet/dry—rate/volume)
- Nausea and vomiting
- Kussmauls (hyperpnea–tachypnea)
- Pulse oximetry
- Barrel chest
- Volume of breath
- Pain, nature of:
  - Pressure (squeezing)
  - Sharp
  - Mild/dull
  - Sudden/slow onset
  - Radiation of pain
  - Location of pain
  - Duration of pain
  - Distant lung sounds
- Cheyne–Stokes (increase–apnea–increase)
- Pain associated with inspiration

Skin color and temperature:

- Cyanosis
- Redness
- Yellow
- Mottling
- Turgor
- Diaphoresis: extreme, mild, moderate
- Warm/dry
- Warm/wet
- Cool/dry
- Cool/wet
- Hot/dry
- Hot/wet

Pupils:

- Equal and reactive to light
- Glaucoma
- Pupils: pinpoint, midsize, dilated, symmetric, round, constricted
- Cataracts
- Contacts
- Sclera: petechiae jaundiced, bloodshot
- Conjunctiva: pale, inflamed, red, lack of tears

Level of consciousness:

- Easily aroused
- Alert and oriented to person, place, and time
- Appropriate words
- Inappropriate behavior
- Confused
- Obeys commands
- Spontaneous eye opening
- Level of sensation

Ability to move:

- Seizure activity: postictal, grand mal, focal
- Ability to discriminate sharp/dull and sensation
- Flexation/extension
- Grip strength
- Pain upon movement

Trauma-related cases:

- Subcutanous emphysema
- Discolored region
- Chest region cyanotic
- Battle's sign
- Swollen tongue
- Distant lung sounds
- Deformity
- Tracheal deviation
- Raccoon eyes
- Flail chest section
- Engorged neck veins
- Jugular distension

- Muffled heart sounds
- Mechanism of injury
- Extreme pain
- Ability to move above and below injury site
- Posturing: decorticate/decerebrate
- Singed lips, nares, and mouth
- Muscle tone
- Pain sharp, dull, burning
- Percent burn

CALL INCIDENT APPROACH

Here I have divided the approach into a call-received format. It is geared to how most of us think while enroute to an incident. The approach is seen as four basic areas of reporting:

Subjective: the history of the patient.
Objective: the head-to-toe assessment.
Assessment: possible problems and other considerations.
Plan: the action taken.

The subjective approach is the one used most widely; it incorporates two ideas in an effective report-writing style.

1. It organizes your thoughts into a basic format.
2. It lends itself to an easy retrieval of thoughts, observations, and the treatment applied.

S: The subjective area is further divided into three categories:
1. Immediate history
2. Pain type and location.
3. Any precipitating events.

O: The objective is a category in which you, the rescuer, have found a problem, an observation. It is made up primarily of a primary and a secondary survey: the head-to-toe assessment along with a mini-neurological examination.

A: The assessment is not a diagnosis but rather possible problems and considerations, be it disease or injury. It is a name attached to a group of signs and symptoms, a possible explanation of what is happening. It should be thought of as an area in which objective findings lead to a possible conclusion. It also provides an area for documentation of observations that do not fit well within textbook cases.

P: This is a plan or action(s) taken. It is brief, concise, yet descriptive comment on the skills used, service rendered, and transportation (i.e., the name of the receiving medical institution). In general it lists the vitals taken, oxygen given and how much, EKG, and so on. Sometimes the report that is provided has an area designed for this type of information. However, if it does not, you must document all skills and procedures applied to the patient.

Cardiac / Chest Pain / Shortness of Breath / CVA / TIA

Subjective: History of the patient:

History of smoking	Prior cardiac/respiratory
Hypotension	Hypertension
Emphysema	Asthma
COPD	Diabetes
Medications/allergies	Headaches

Pain/Type/Locations	*Precipitating events*
Sharp pain	Activity before the event
Dull pain	Activity after the event
Radiating pain	Incident with or without activity
Crushing pain	Location of the patient before
Chest	Location of patient after
Back	Exposure to an unusual event
Side(s)	Patient found/position/area
Arm(s)	
Leg(s)	
Head	

Objective: Head-to-toe assessment (see "Head-to-Toe Approach"):

Pupils	Level of consciousness
Sclera	Skin color/temperature
Conjunctiva	Vitals: B/P, P, R
Facial tone	Heart sounds
Neck musculature	Mini-neurological assessment
Adequate	Oriented to person, place, time
ventilations	Pupils, posture
Rales–rhonchi–stridor	Level of consciousness
Wheezing–snoring	Capillary refill
Distant sounds	Glasgow coma score
Extremities	Ability to move
Grip strength	Orthostatic B/P
Distal pulse	Pulse oximetry
Flexation/extension	
Abdominal status	
Point tenderness	
Rebound–rigid	

Assessment: Possible problems and other considerations:

Cardiac disease	Respiratory disease
CVA	TIA
Arrhythmia	Head injury
Tension pneumothorax	Asthma
	Emphysema
Congential history	COPD
Trauma (see the Auto and GSW sections)	Croup
	Pulmonary embolism
	Aortic aneurysm

Environmental exposure	Pleurisy
Pericarditis	
Vaso/vagal reaction	
Epiglotitis	

Plan: Action taken, skills performed:

Procedure		*Response*
Airway		
Oropharyngea	• Time placed/who placed • Size used • Supplemental oxygen • Adjunctive equipment	• Skin color/temperature • Breath sounds • Capillary refill • Chest expansion
Esophageal	• Time placed/who placed • Supplemental oxygen • Adjunctive equipment	• Skin color/temperature • Breath sounds • Capillary refill • Chest expansion • Gastric distension
Endotracheal	• Time placed/who placed • Size used • Tube passed with cord visualization • Oral/nasal introduction	• Skin color/temperature • Breath sounds • Capillary refill • Chest expansion • Epigastric silent • Gastric distension
Suctioning	• Oral/tracheal • Time/who suctioned	• Fluid evacuated • Capillary refill • Skin color/temperature • Mental status
Breathing		
Oxygen	• Device used • Time/who applied • Liter flow • Adjunctive equipment	• Skin color/temperature • Capillary refill • Patient position • Mental status • Mucosa color
BVM/demand	• Time/who applied • Adjunctive equipment	• Skin color • Chest expansion • Gastric distension
Pulse oximetry	• Time/who applied • Type of probe	• Percent oxygen saturation
Circulation		
CPR/mechanical	• Time started	• Pulse present with compression
Monitor	• Time/who applied • Lead placed	• Skin color/temperature • Breath sounds

	• EKG interpretation	• Before and after all treatments and medications
IV	• Time/who placed • Size of cathcter • Location of IV • Fluid type	• Blood drawn • Vitals
Defib./cardio.	• Time/who placed • Watts/second used	• EKG response, before and after
External pace	• Time/who placed • Milliampere rate	• EKG response, before and after
Drug admin.	• Time/who placed • Drug type • Dosage • Route: SQ, IM, IV, ETT	• Mental status • EKG response • Vital response • Pain relief

Auto / Motorcycle / Bicycle Accident / Pedestrian

Subjective: History of the patient:

General history
Hypotension
Emphysema
COPD
Medications/allergies
Hemophilletic
Child restraint
Seatbelts on
Hypertension
Asthma
Diabetes
Headaches
Helmet

Pain / Type / Locations

Sharp pain
Dull pain
Radiating pain
Crushing pain
Chest–abdomen
Back–head
Side(s)
Arm(s)
Leg(s)
Head

Precipitating events

Activity before the event
Activity after the event
Approximate time of the incident
Location of patient before
Location of patient after
Type of accident
Point of impact
Patient found/position
Type/number of vehicles

Objective: Head-to-toe assessment (see "Head-to-Toe Approach"):

Pupils
Sclera
Conjunctiva
Facial tone
Nose, ears, and mouth
Neck musculature
Chest integrity
Level of consciousness
Skin color/temperature
Vitals: B/P, P, R
Crepitus: raccoon eyes
CNS/blood: Battle's sign
Tracheal deviation
Paradoxical breathing
Heart sounds

Adequate ventilations
- Rales–rhonchi–stridor
- Wheezing–snoring
- Distant sounds

Extremities
- Grip strength
- Distal pulse
- Flexation/extension

Obvious hemorrhaging
Pelvic integrity
Abdominal status
- Point–Rebound–Rigid

Mini-neurological assessment
- Oriented to person, place, time
- Pupils, posture
- Level of consciousness

Capillary refill
Glasgow coma score
Ability to move
Bleeding rectally
Pulse oximetry
Bleeding vaginally
Trauma score

Assessment: Possible problems and other considerations:

Cardiac disease
CVA
Arrhythmia
Tension pneumothorax
Congential history
Trauma (see the Auto and GSW sections)
Environmental exposure
Pericarditis
Vaso/vagal reaction
Swollen tongue
Discolored region
Insulin reaction
Respiratory disease
TIA
Head injury
Asthma
Emphysema
COPD
Flail chest
Pulmonary embolism
Aortic aneurysm
Muffled heart tones
If pregnant, fetal heart tones (see the Obstetrics section)

Plan: Action taken, skills performed:

Procedure		*Response*
Airway		
Oropharyngeal	• Time placed/who placed • Size used • Supplemental oxygen • Adjunctive equipment	• Skin color/temperature • Breath sounds • Capillary refill • Chest expansion
Esophageal	• Time placed/who placed • Supplemental oxygen • Adjunctive equipment	• Skin color/temperature • Breath sounds • Capillary refill • Chest expansion • Gastric distension
Endotracheal	• Time placed/who placed • Size used • Tube passed with cord visualization • Oral/nasal introduction	• Skin color/temperature • Breath sounds • Capillary refill • Chest expansion • Epigastric silent • Gastric distension

Suctioning	• Oral/tracheal • Time/who suctioned	• Fluid evacuated • Capillary refill • Skin color/temperature • Mental status
Cervical Spinal	• Device used Cervical collar Cervical immobilization Blanket roll KED/backboard • Time device applied • Adjunctive equipment	• Extremity pulses • Sensations • Capillary refill • Skin color/temperature • Mechanism of injury • Mini-neurological assessment before/after
Breathing		
Oxygen	• Device used • Time/who applied • Liter flow • Adjunctive equipment	• Skin color/temperature • Capillary refill • Patient position • Mental status • Mucosa color
BVM/demand	• Time/who applied • Adjunctive equipment	• Skin color • Chest expansion • Gastric distension
Pulse oximetry	• Time/who applied • Type of probe	• Percent oxygen saturation
Circulation		
CPR/mechanical	• Time started	• Pulse present with compression
Monitor	• Time/who applied • Lead placed • EKG interpretation	• Skin color/temperature • Breath sounds • Before and after all treatments and medications
IV	• Time/who placed • Size of catheter • Location of IV • Fluid type	• Blood drawn • Vitals
Defib./cardio.	• Time/who placed • Watts/second used	• EKG response, before and after
External pace	• Time/who placed • Milliampere rate	• EKG response, before and after
Drug admin.	• Time/who placed • Drug type • Dosage • Route: SQ, IM, IV, ETT	• Mental status • EKG response • Vital response • Pain relief

MAST	• Time/who placed • Sections inflated • Adjunctive equipment	• Extremity pulses • Capillary refill • Mental status
Hemorrhage Bandage/ dressing	• Time/who placed • Pressure points used • Direct pressure used • Type dressing applied • Location of splint • Adjunctive equipment	• Extremity pulses • Estimated blood loss • Capillary refill • Skin color/temperature • Sensation

SUICIDE / PSYCHOLOGICAL / ALCOHOL / SUBSTANCE ABUSE / OD / POISONING

Subjective: History of the patient:

General History
Hypotension
Emphysema
COPD
Medications/allergies
Hemophilletic
Prior substance abuse
Prior alcohol abuse

Prior cardiac disease
Hypertension
Asthma
Diabetes
Headaches
AIDS
Prior attempts at suicide
Psychological history

Pain / Type / Locations

Sharp pain
Dull pain
Radiating pain
Crushing pain
Chest–abdomen
Back–head
Side(s)
Arm(s)
Leg(s)
Head
Type of suicide:
- GSW
- Hanging
- Medication OD
- Other

Precipitating events

Activity before the event
Activity after the event
Approximate time of the incident
Location of patient before
Location of patient after
Type of incident
Exposure to unusual event
Patient found/position
Patient spoke about: wish to die, wants relief from suffering; recent divorce, separation, death, failing health, financial problems

Objective: Head-to-toe assessment: (see "Head-to-Toe Approach"):

Pupils
Sclera
Conjunctiva
Facial tone
Nose, ears, and mouth
Neck musculature
Chest integrity
Adequate ventilations
- Rales–rhonchi–stridor
- Wheezing–snoring
- Distant sounds

Extremities
- Grip strength

Level of consciousness
Skin color/temperature
Vitals: B/P: P, R
Crepitus/raccoon eyes
CNS/blood: Battle's sign
Tracheal deviation
Paradoxal breathing
Heart sounds
Mini-neurological assessment
- Oriented to person, place, time
- Pupils, posture
- Level of consciousness

Capillary refill

Distal pulse	Glasgow coma score
Flexation/extension	Ability to move
Obvious hemorrhaging	Bleeding rectally
Pelvic integrity	Pulse oximetry
Abdominal status	Bleeding vaginally
Point–rebound–rigid	Trauma score

Assessment: Possible problems and other considerations:

Cardiac disease	Respiratory disease
CVA	TIA
Arrhythmia	Head injury

Note the presence of all persons.
If deceased, note the position of the body.
Control the scene until police arrive.
If there is a possibility of scene violence, stage until the police can control the scene.

Plan: Action taken, skills performed:

Procedure		*Response*
Airway		
Oropharyngeal	• Time placed/who placed • Size used • Supplemental oxygen • Adjunctive equipment	• Skin color/temperature • Breath sounds • Capillary refill • Chest expansion
Esophageal	• Time placed/who placed • Supplemental oxygen • Adjunctive equipment	• Skin color/temperature • Breath sounds • Capillary refill • Chest expansion • Gastric distension
Endotracheal	• Time placed/who placed • Size used • Tube passed with cord visualization • Oral/nasal introduction	• Skin color/temperature • Breath sounds • Capillary refill • Chest expansion • Epigastric silent • Gastric distension
Suctioning	• Oral/tracheal • Time/who suctioned	• Fluid evacuated • Capillary refill • Skin color/temperature • Mental status
Cervical Spinal	• Device used Cervical collar Cervical immobilization Blanket roll KED/backboard	• Extremity pulses • Sensations • Capillary refill • Skin color/temperature

	• Time device applied • Adjunctive equipment	• Mechanism of injury • Mini-neurological assessment before/after
Breathing		
Oxygen	• Device used • Time/who applied • Liter flow • Adjunctive equipment	• Skin color/temperature • Capillary refill • Patient position • Mental status • Mucosa color
BVM/demand	• Time/who applied • Adjunctive equipment	• Skin color • Chest expansion • Gastric distension
Pulse oximetry	• Time/who applied • Type of probe	• Percent oxygen saturation
Circulation		
CPR/mechanical	• Time started	• Pulse present with compression
Monitor	• Time/who applied • Lead placed • EKG interpretation	• Skin color/temperature • Breath sounds • Before and after all treatments and medications
IV	• Time/who placed • Size of catheter • Location of IV • Fluid type	• Blood drawn • Vitals
Defib./cardio.	• Time/who placed • Watts/second used	• EKG response, before and after
External pace	• Time/who placed • Milliampere rate	• EKG response, before and after
Drug admin.	• Time/who placed • Drug type • Dosage • Route: SQ, IM, IV, ETT	• Mental status • EKG response • Vital response • Pain relief
MAST	• Time/who placed • Sections inflated • Adjunctive equipment	• Extremity pulses • Capillary refill • Mental status
Hemorrhage		
Bandage/dressing	• Time/who placed • Pressure points used • Direct pressure used • Type dressing applied • Location of splint • Adjunctive equipment	• Extremity pulses • Estimated blood loss • Capillary refill • Skin color/temperature • Sensation

Diabetic / Hypoglycemic Event / Seizure

Subjective: History of the patient:

History of smoking
Hypotension
Emphysema
COPD
Medications/allergies
Headaches
Recent surgery
Prior cardiac/respiratory
Hypertension
Asthma
Diabetes
- Diet controlled
- Insulin dependent
- Type of insulin (NPH, REG)

Seizure activity
Type of seizure
- Full body, focal

Neurological history

Pain / Type / Locations

Sharp pain
Dull pain
Radiating pain
Crushing pain
Chest
Back
Side(s)
Arm(s)
Leg(s)
Head

Precipitating events

Activity before the event
Activity after the event
Incident with or without activity
Location of patient before
Location of patient after
Exposure to an unusual event
Patient found/position/area

Objective: Head-to-toe assessment (see "Head-to-Toe Approach"):

Pupils
Sclera
Conjunctiva
Facial tone
Neck musculature
Adequate ventilations
- Rales–rhonchi–stridor
- Wheezing–snoring
- Distant sounds

Extremities
- Grip strength
- Distal pulse
- Flexation/extension

Abdominal status
- Point tenderness
- Rebound–rigid

Level of consciousness
Skin color/temperature
Vitals: B/P, P, R
Heart sounds
Mini-neurological assessment
- Oriented to person, place, time
- Pupils, posture
- Level of consciousness

Capillary refill
Glasgow coma score
Ability to move
Orthostatic B/P
Pulse oximetry

Assessment: Possible problems and other considerations:

Cardiac disease
CVA
Arrhythmia
Tension pneumothorax
Respiratory disease
TIA
Head injury
Asthma
Emphysema

Congential history
Trauma (see the Auto and GSW sections)
Environmental exposure
Pericarditis
Vaso/vagal reaction
Epiglotitis
Drug overdose
Alcohol ingestion
COPD
Croup
Pulmonary embolism
Aortic aneurysm
Pleurisy
Insulin not taken
Poor diet

Plan: Action taken, skills performed:

	Procedure	*Response*
Airway		
Oropharyngeal	• Time placed/who placed • Size used • Supplemental oxygen • Adjunctive equipment	• Skin color/temperature • Breath sounds • Capillary refill • Chest expansion
Esophageal	• Time placed/who placed • Supplemental oxygen • Adjunctive equipment	• Skin color/temperature • Breath sounds • Capillary refill • Chest expansion • Gastric distension
Endotracheal	• Time placed/who placed • Size used • Tube passed with cord visualization • Oral/nasal introduction	• Skin color/temperature • Breath sounds • Capillary refill • Chest expansion • Epigastric silent • Gastric distension
Suctioning	• Oral/tracheal • Time/who suctioned	• Fluid evacuated • Capillary refill • Skin color/temperature • Mental status
Breathing		
Oxygen	• Device used • Time/who applied • Liter flow • Adjunctive equipment	• Skin color/temperature • Capillary refill • Patient position • Mental status • Mucosa color
BVM/demand	• Time/who applied • Adjunctive equipment	• Skin color • Chest expansion • Gastric distension
Pulse oximetry	• Time/who applied • Type of probe	• Percent oxygen saturation
Circulation		
CPR/mechanical	• Time started	• Pulse present with compression

Monitor	• Time/who applied • Lead placed • EKG interpretation	• Skin color/temperature • Breath sounds • Before and after all treatments and medications
IV	• Time/who placed • Size of catheter • Location of IV • Fluid type	• Blood drawn • Vitals
Defib./cardio.	• Time/who placed • Watts/second used	• EKG response, before and after
External pace	• Time/who placed • Milliampere rate	• EKG response, before and after
Drug admin.	• Time/who placed • Drug type • Dosage • Route: SQ, IM, IV, ETT	• Mental status • EKG response • Vital response • Pain relief

GSW / Assault / Fall

Subjective: History of the patient:

General history
Hypotension
Type of assault
  Battery
  Sexual
  Molestation
Child/geriatric abuse
Medications/allergies

Distance from the weapon
Hypertension
Description of the weapon
Type of weapon
Ammunition used (caliber)
Fall distance noted
All wounds noted, head to toe
Recent hospitalization

Pain / Type / Locations

Sharp pain
Dull pain
Radiating pain
Crushing pain
Chest–abdomen
Back–head
Side(s)
Arm(s)
Leg(s)
Head

Precipitating events

Activity before the event
Activity after the event
Approximate time of the incident
Location of patient before
Location of patient after
Type of accident
Point of impact
Patient found/position
Drugs (contraband) present

Objective: Head-to-toe assessment (see "Head-to-Toe Approach"):

Pupils
Sclera
Conjunctiva
Facial tone
Nose, ears, and mouth
Neck musculature

Level of consciousness
Skin color/temperature
Vitals: B/P, P, R
Crepitus: raccoon eyes
CNS/blood: Battle's sign
Tracheal deviation
Paradoxical breathing

- Chest integrity
- Adequate ventilations
  - Rales–rhonchi–stridor
  - Wheezing–snoring
  - Distant sounds
- Extremities
  - Grip strength
  - Distal pulse
  - Flexation/extension
- Obvious hemorrhage
- Pelvic integrity
- Abdominal status
  - Point–rebound–rigid
- Heart sounds
- Mini-neurological assessment
  - Oriented to person, place, time
  - Pupils, posture
  - Level of consciousness
- Capillary refill
- Glasgow coma score
- Ability to move
- Bleeding rectally
- Pulse oximetry
- Entrance/exit wounds
- Bleeding vaginally
- Trauma score

Assessment: Possible problems and other considerations:

- Arrhythmia
- Tension pneumothorax
- Congential history
- Trauma (see the Auto and GSW sections)
- Environmental exposure
- Muffled heart tones
- Head injury
- Flail chest
- Emphysema
- COPD
- If pregnant, fetal heart tones (see the Obstetrics section)

Plan: Action taken, skills performed:

Procedure		*Response*
Airway		
Oropharyngeal	• Time placed/who placed • Size used • Supplemental oxygen • Adjunctive equipment	• Skin color/temperature • Breath sounds • Capillary refill • Chest expansion
Esophageal	• Time placed/who placed • Supplemental oxygen • Adjunctive equipment	• Skin color/temperature • Breath sounds • Capillary refill • Chest expansion • Gastric distension
Endotracheal	• Time placed/who placed • Size used • Tube passed with cord visualization • Oral/nasal introduction	• Skin color/temperature • Breath sounds • Capillary refill • Chest expansion • Epigastric silent • Gastric distension
Suctioning	• Oral/tracheal • Time/who suctioned	• Fluid evacuated • Capillary refill • Skin color/temperature • Mental status

Cervical Spinal	• Device used Cervical collar Cervical immobilization Blanket roll KED/backboard • Time device applied • Adjunctive equipment	• Extremity pulses • Sensations • Capillary refill • Skin color/temperature • Mechanism of injury • Mini-neurological assessment before/after
Breathing Oxygen	• Device used • Time/who applied • Liter flow • Adjunctive equipment	• Skin color/temperature • Capillary refill • Patient position • Mental status • Mucosa color
BVM/demand	• Time/who applied • Adjunctive equipment	• Skin color • Chest expansion • Gastric distension
Pulse oximetry	• Time/who applied • Type of probe	• Percent oxygen saturation
Circulation CPR/mechanical	• Time started	• Pulse present with compression
Monitor	• Time/who applied • Lead placed • EKG interpretation	• Skin color/temperature • Breath sounds • Before and after all treatments and medications
IV	• Time/who placed • Size of catheter • Location of IV • Fluid type	• Blood drawn • Vitals
Defib./cardio.	• Time/who placed • Watts/second used	• EKG response, before and after
External pace	• Time/who placed • Milliampere rate	• EKG response, before and after
Drug admin.	• Time/who placed • Drug type • Dosage • Route: SQ, IM, IV, ETT	• Mental status • EKG response • Vital response • Pain relief
MAST	• Time/who placed • Sections inflated • Adjunctive equipment	• Extremity pulses • Capillary refill • Mental status

Hemorrhage

Bandage/dressing
- Time/who placed
- Pressure points used
- Direct pressure used
- Type dressing applied
- Location of splint
- Adjunctive equipment
- Extremity pulses
- Estimated blood loss
- Capillary refill
- Skin color/temperature
- Sensation

FIRE / BURN / ELECTRICAL SHOCK

Subjective: History of the patient:

General history
Hypotension
Hypertension
COPD
Medications/allergies
Electrical source
  Know current source/amount
  Potential additional injury

Type of fire involvement
  House fire
  Chemical fire
Environmental
  Confinement
  Explosion
  Hazardous material

Pain/Type/Locations

Sharp pain
Dull pain
Radiating pain
Crushing pain
Chest–abdomen
Back–head
Side(s)
Arm(s)
Leg(s)
Head

Precipitating events

Activity before the event
Activity after the event
Approximate time of the incident
Location of patient before
Location of patient after
Type of incident
Exposure to unusual event
Patient found/position
Safety equipment used

Objective: Head-to-toe assessment (see "Head-to-Toe Approach"):

Pupils
Sclera
Conjunctiva
Facial tone
Nose, ears, and mouth
Neck musculature
Chest integrity
Adequate ventilations
  Rales–rhonchi–stridor
  Wheezing–snoring
  Distant sounds
Extremities
  Grip strength
  Distal pulse
  Flexation/extension
Obvious hemorrhage

Level of consciousness
Skin color/temperature
Vitals: B/P, P, R
Crepitus: raccoon eyes
CNS/blood: Battle's sign
Tracheal deviation
Paradoxical breathing
Heart sounds
Mini-neurological assessment
  Oriented to person, place, time
  Pupils, posture
  Level of consciousness
Capillary refill
Glasgow coma score
Ability to move
Bleeding rectally
Pulse oximetry

Pelvic integrity
Abdominal status
  Point–rebound–rigid
Mechanism of injury
  Type burn
  Explosion shock wave
  Chemical burn

Bleeding vaginally
Trauma score
Burns present
  Degree of burn
  Body area involvement
  Respiratory involvement
  Causative agent

Assessment: Possible problems and other considerations:

If hazardous materials involved (See Chapter 3)
  Type of chemical
  UN/DOT number
  Wind direction
  Ambient air temperature/humidity
Respiratory involvement
  Nares checked
  Lungs checked
Oral cavity checked

Plan: Action taken, skills performed:

Procedure		*Response*
Airway		
Oropharyngeal	• Time placed/who placed • Size used • Supplemental oxygen • Adjunctive equipment	• Skin color/temperature • Breath sounds • Capillary refill • Chest expansion
Esophageal	• Time placed/who placed • Supplemental oxygen • Adjunctive equipment	• Skin color/temperature • Breath sounds • Capillary refill • Chest expansion • Gastric distension
Endotracheal	• Time placed/who placed • Size used • Tube passed with cord visualization • Oral/nasal introduction	• Skin color/temperature • Breath sounds • Capillary refill • Chest expansion • Epigastric silent • Gastric distension
Suctioning	• Oral/tracheal • Time/who suctioned	• Fluid evacuated • Capillary refill • Skin color/temperature • Mental status
Cervical		
Spinal	• Device used Cervical collar Cervical immobilization Blanket roll KED/backboard	• Extremity pulses • Sensations • Capillary refill • Skin color/temperature

	Chapter 4	Assessment Report Categories
	• Time device applied • Adjunctive equipment	• Mechanism of injury • Mini-neurological assessment before/after
Breathing		
Oxygen	• Device used • Time/who applied • Liter flow • Adjunctive equipment	• Skin color/temperature • Capillary refill • Patient position • Mental status • Mucosa color
BVM/demand	• Time/who applied • Adjunctive equipment	• Skin color • Chest expansion • Gastric distension
Pulse oximetry	• Time/who applied • Type of probe	• Percent oxygen saturation
Circulation		
CPR/mechanical	• Time started	• Pulse present with compression
Monitor	• Time/who applied • Lead placed • EKG interpretation	• Skin color/temperature • Breath sounds • Before and after all treatments and medications
IV	• Time/who placed • Size of catheter • Location of IV • Fluid type	• Blood drawn • Vitals
Defib./cardio.	• Time/who placed • Watts/second used	• EKG response, before and after
External pace	• Time/who placed • Milliampere rate	• EKG response, before and after
Drug admin.	• Time/who placed • Drug type • Dosage • Route: SQ, IM, IV, ETT	• Mental status • EKG response • Vital response • Pain relief
MAST	• Time/who placed • Sections inflated • Adjunctive equipment	• Extremity pulses • Capillary refill • Mental status
Hemorrhage		
Bandage/dressing	• Time/who placed • Pressure points used • Direct pressure used • Type dressing applied • Location of splint • Adjunctive equipment	• Extremity pulses • Estimated blood loss • Capillary refill • Skin color/temperature • Sensation

Splinting	• Time/who placed	• Extremity pulses
	• Type of splint	• Capillary refill
	• Location of splint	• Distal sensation
	• Adjunctive equipment	• Skin color/temperature

Laceration / Abrasion / Amputation / Fracture

Subjective: History of the patient (see the GSW section):

General history	Mechanism of injury
Hypotension	Hypertension
All wounds noted head to toe	
Pain/Type/Locations	*Precipitating events*
Sharp pain	Activity before the event
Dull pain	Activity after the event
Radiating pain	Approximate time of the incident
Crushing pain	Location of patient before
Chest–abdomen	Location of patient after
Back–head	Type of accident
Side(s)	Point of impact
Arm(s)	Patient found/position
Leg(s)	Drugs (contraband) present
Head	

Objective: Head-to-toe assessment (see "Head-to-Toe Approach"):

Pupils	Level of consciousness
Sclera	Skin color/temperature
Conjunctiva	Vitals: B/P, P, R
Facial tone	Crepitus: raccoon eyes
Nose, ears, and mouth	CNS/blood: Battle's sign
Neck musculature	Tracheal deviation
Chest integrity	Paradoxical breathing
Adequate ventilations	Heart sounds
Rales–rhonchi–stridor	Mini-neurological assessment
Wheezing–snoring	Oriented to person, place, time
Distant sounds	Pupils, posture
Extremities	Level of consciousness
Grip strength	Capillary refill
Distal pulse	Glasgow coma score
Flexation/extension	Ability to move
Obvious hemorrhage	Bleeding rectally
Pelvic integrity	Pulse oximetry
Abdominal status	Entrance/exit wounds
Point–rebound–rigid	Bleeding vaginally
	Trauma score

Assessment: Possible problems and other considerations:

Note: Any of the following may be a result of system insult.

Arrhythmia	Head injury
Tension pneumothorax	Flail chest
	Emphysema

Congenital history
Trauma (see the Auto and GSW sections)
Environmental exposure
Muffled heart tones
COPD
If pregnant, fetal heart tones (see the Obstetrics section)

Plan: Action taken, skills performed:

Procedure		*Response*
Airway		
Oropharyngeal	• Time placed/who placed • Size used • Supplemental oxygen • Adjunctive equipment	• Skin color/temperature • Breath sounds • Capillary refill • Chest expansion
Esophageal	• Time placed/who placed • Supplemental oxygen • Adjunctive equipment	• Skin color/temperature • Breath sounds • Capillary refill • Chest expansion • Gastric distension
Endotracheal	• Time placed/who placed • Size used • Tube passed with cord visualization • Oral/nasal introduction	• Skin color/temperature • Breath sounds • Capillary refill • Chest expansion • Epigastric silent • Gastric distension
Suctioning	• Oral/tracheal • Time/who suctioned	• Fluid evacuated • Capillary refill • Skin color/temperature • Mental status
Cervical		
Spinal	• Device used Cervical collar Cervical immobilization Blanket roll KED/backboard • Time device applied • Adjunctive equipment	• Extremity pulses • Sensations • Capillary refill • Skin color/temperature • Mechanism of injury • Mini-neurological assessment before/after
Breathing		
Oxygen	• Device used • Time/who applied • Liter flow • Adjunctive equipment	• Skin color/temperature • Capillary refill • Patient position • Mental status • Mucosa color
BVM/demand	• Time/who applied • Adjunctive equipment	• Skin color • Chest expansion • Gastric distension

Pulse oximetry	• Time/who applied • Type of probe	• Percent oxygen saturation
Circulation		
CPR/mechanical	• Time started	• Pulse present with compression
Monitor	• Time/who applied • Lead placed • EKG interpretation	• Skin color/temperature • Breath sounds • Before and after all treatments and medications
IV	• Time/who placed • Size of catheter • Location of IV • Fluid type	• Blood drawn • Vitals
Defib./cardio.	• Time/who placed • Watts/second used	• EKG response, before and after
External pace	• Time/who placed • Milliampere rate	• EKG response, before and after
Drug admin.	• Time/who placed • Drug type • Dosage • Route: SQ, IM, IV, ETT	• Mental status • EKG response • Vital response • Pain relief
MAST	• Time/who placed • Sections inflated • Adjunctive equipment	• Extremity pulses • Capillary refill • Mental status
Hemorrhage		
Bandage/dressing	• Time/who placed • Pressure points used • Direct pressure used • Type dressing applied • Location of splint • Adjunctive equipment	• Extremity pulses • Estimated blood loss • Capillary refill • Skin color/temperature • Sensation
Splinting	• Time/who placed • Type of splint • Location of splint • Adjunctive equipment • Amputated body part placed on ice	• Extremity pulses • Capillary refill • Distal sensation • Skin color/temperature

Near-Drowning / Diving Accident

Subjective: History of the patient:

General history
Area surrounding the event

SCUBA:
Depth, time down, surface
Type of diving: skin/SCUBA

Swimming pool
Pond, lake
River, stream
Two-point triangulation

Diving alone, distance from nearest diver, under instruction, cave diving, night dive, diver's experience

Pain/Type/Locations

Sharp pain
Dull pain
Radiating pain
Crushing pain
Chest
Back
Side(s)
Arm(s)
Leg(s)
Head
Pain in joints

Precipitating events

Activity before the event
Activity after the event
Incident with or without activity
Location of patient before
Location of patient after
Exposure to an unusual event
Patient found/position area
Medications/allergies

Objective: Head-to-toe assessment (see "Head-to-Toe Approach"):

Pupils
Sclera
Conjunctiva
Facial tone
Neck musculature
Adequate ventilations
- Rales–rhonchi–stridor
- Wheezing–snoring
- Distant sounds

- Extremities
  - Grip strength
  - Distal pulse
  - Flexation/extension
- Abdominal status
  - Point tenderness
  - Rebound–rigid

Level of consciousness
Skin color/temperature
Vitals: B/P, P, R
Heart sounds
Mini-neurological assessment
- Oriented to person, place, time
- Pupils, posture
- Level of consciousness

Capillary refill
Glasgow coma score
Ability to move
Orthostatic B/P
Pulse oximetry

Assessment: Possible problems and other considerations:

Cardiac arrhythmia
CVA
Itching with/without rash
Tension pneumothorax
Dizziness: history
Staggering gait
Pulmonary embolism
Hearing defect
Tinnitus

Respiratory difficulty
TIA
Head injury
Mediastinal emphysema
Subcutaneous emphysema
Convulsions
Environmental exposure
Pulmonary embolism

Plan: Action taken, skills performed:

Procedure		*Response*
Airway		
Oropharyngeal	• Time placed/who placed • Size used • Supplemental oxygen • Adjunctive equipment	• Skin color/temperature • Breath sounds • Capillary refill • Chest expansion
Esophageal	• Time placed/who placed • Supplemental oxygen • Adjunctive equipment	• Skin color/temperature • Breath sounds • Capillary refill • Chest expansion • Gastric distension
Endotracheal	• Time placed/who placed • Size used • Tube passed with cord visualization • Oral/nasal introduction	• Skin color/temperature • Breath sounds • Capillary refill • Chest expansion • Epigastric silent • Gastric distension
Suctioning	• Oral/tracheal • Time/who suctioned	• Fluid evacuated • Capillary refill • Skin color/temperature • Mental status
Breathing		
Oxygen	• Device used • Time/who applied • Liter flow • Adjunctive equipment	• Skin color/temperature • Capillary refill • Patient position • Mental status • Mucosa color
BVM/demand	• Time/who applied • Adjunctive equipment	• Skin color • Chest expansion • Gastric distension
Pulse oximetry	• Time/who applied • Type of probe	• Percent oxygen saturation
Circulation		
CPR/mechanical	• Time started	• Pulse present with compression
Monitor	• Time/who applied • Lead placed • EKG interpretation	• Skin color/temperature • Breath sounds • Before and after all treatments and medications

IV	• Time/who placed • Size of catheter • Location of IV • Fluid type	• Blood drawn • Vitals
Defib./cardio.	• Time/who placed • Watts/second used	• EKG response, before and after
External pace	• Time/who placed • Milliampere rate	• EKG response, before and after
Drug admin.	• Time/who placed • Drug type • Dosage • Route: SQ, IM, IV, ETT	• Mental status • EKG response • Vital response • Pain relief
MAST	• Time/who placed • Sections inflated • Adjunctive equipment	• Extremity pulses • Capillary refill • Mental status
Hemorrhage Bandage/dressing	• Time/who placed • Pressure points used • Direct pressure used • Type dressing applied • Location of splint • Adjunctive equipment	• Extremity pulses • Estimated blood loss • Capillary refill • Skin color/temperature • Sensation
Splinting	• Time/who placed • Type of splint • Location of splint • Adjunctive equipment	• Extremity pulses • Capillary refill • Distal sensation • Skin color/temperature
Transportation	• Patient placed in high Trendelenburg position • Low-level flight if aircraft is used, below 500 feet • Establish communication with recompression chamber	

Obstetrics / Gynecology / Neonate

Subjective: History of the patient: (see "Body Systems Approach—Reproductive System"):

General history	Prior cardiac/respiratory
Hypotension	Hypertension
Prenatal care/education	Length of present pregnancy
	Previous live births

- Month of conception
- Vaginal discharge:
  - clear/bloody/clots
- Pedal edema
- Polyuria
- Syncopal episode
- Medications/allergies
- Abortions/miscarriages
- Abnormal:
  - Eclampsia
  - Toxemia
  - Placenta previa
  - Placenta abrupto

Pain/Type/Locations

- Sharp pain
- Dull pain
- Radiating pain
- Crushing pain
- Chest–abdomen
- Back–head
- Side(s)
- Arm(s)
- Leg(s)
- Head

Precipitating events

- Activity before the event
- Activity after the event
- Approximate time of the incident
- Location of patient before
- Location of patient after
- Patient found/position/area

Objective: Head-to-toe assessment (see "Head-to-Toe Approach"):

- Pupils
- Sclera
- Conjunctiva
- Facial tone
- Nose, ears, and mouth
- Neck musculature
- Chest integrity
- Adequate ventilations
  - Rales–rhonchi–stridor
  - Wheezing–snoring
  - Distant sounds
- Extremities
  - Grip strength
  - Distal pulse
  - Flexation/extension
  - Obvious hemorrhage
  - Pelvic integrity
  - Abdominal status
    - Point–rebound–rigid
  - Time of birth
- Level of consciousness
- Skin color/temperature
- Vitals: B/P, P, R
- Raccoon eyes
- CNS/blood: Battle's sign
- Merconium staining
- Seizure activity
- Heart sounds
- Mini-neurological assessment
  - Oriented to person, place, time
  - Pupils, posture
  - Level of consciousness
- Capillary refill
- Glasgow coma score
- Ability to move
- Bleeding rectally
- Pulse oximetry
- Fetal/neonatal heart sounds
- Bleeding vaginally
- Trauma score

Assessment: Possible problems and other considerations:

- Merconium aspiration
- Prolapsed cord
- Congenital history
- Ectopic pregnancy
- Multiple births
- Umbilical presentation
- Respiratory distress
- Ruptured uterus
- Premature birth
- Incomplete delivery
- Breech delivery
- Trauma (see the Auto and GSW sections)
- Environmental exposure

Respiratory (see the Cardiac section)	APGAR score
Muffled heart tones	

Plan: Action taken, skills performed:

Procedure		*Response*
Airway		
Oropharyngeal	• Time placed/who placed • Size used • Supplemental oxygen • Adjunctive equipment	• Skin color/temperature • Breath sounds • Capillary refill • Chest expansion
Esophageal	• Time placed/who placed • Supplemental oxygen • Adjunctive equipment	• Skin color/temperature • Breath sounds • Capillary refill • Chest expansion • Gastric distension
Endotracheal	• Time placed/who placed • Size used • Tube passed with cord visualization • Oral/nasal introduction	• Skin color/temperature • Breath sounds • Capillary refill • Chest expansion • Epigastric silent • Gastric distension
Suctioning	• Oral/tracheal • Time/who suctioned	• Fluid evacuated • Capillary refill • Skin color/temperature • Mental status
Cervical		
Spinal	• Device used Cervical collar Cervical immobilization Blanket roll KED/backboard • Time device applied • Adjunctive equipment	• Extremity pulses • Sensations • Capillary refill • Skin color/temperature • Mechanism of injury • Mini-neurological assessment: before/after
Breathing		
Oxygen	• Device used • Time/who applied • Liter flow • Adjunctive equipment	• Skin color/temperature • Capillary refill • Patient position • Mental status • Mucosa color
BVM/demand	• Time/who applied • Adjunctive equipment	• Skin color • Chest expansion • Gastric distension
Pulse oximetry	• Time/who applied • Type of probe	• Percent oxygen saturation

Circulation		
CPR/mechanical	• Time started	• Pulse present with compression
Monitor	• Time/who applied • Lead placed • EKG interpretation	• Skin color/temperature • Breath sounds • Before and after all treatments and medications
IV	• Time/who placed • Size of catheter • Location of IV • Fluid type	• Blood drawn • Vitals
Defib./cardio.	• Time/who placed • Watts/second used	• EKG response, before and after
External pace	• Time/who placed • Milliampere rate	• EKG response, before and after
Drug admin.	• Time/who placed • Drug type • Dosage • Route: SQ, IM, IV, ETT	• Mental status • EKG response • Vital response • Pain relief
MAST	• Time/who placed • Sections inflated • Adjunctive equipment	• Extremity pulses • Capillary refill • Mental status
Hemorrhage		
Bandage/dressing	• Time/who placed • Pressure points used • Direct pressure used • Type dressing applied • Location of splint • Adjunctive equipment	• Extremity pulses • Estimated blood loss • Capillary refill • Skin color/temperature • Sensation

General Illness

Subjective: History of the patient:

General history	Asthma/emphysema
Hypotension	Diabetes
Hypertension	Headaches
COPD	Medications
Seizure activity	Allergies
Pain/Type/Locations	*Precipitating events*
Sharp pain	Activity before the event
Dull pain	Activity after the event
Radiating pain	Approximate time of the incident
Crushing pain	Location of patient before

Chest–abdomen
Back–head
Side(s)
Arm(s)
Leg(s)
Head

Location of patient after
Type of incident
Exposure to unusual event
Patient found/position

Objective: Head-to-toe assessment (see "Head-to-Toe Approach"):

Pupils
Sclera
Conjunctiva
Facial tone
Nose, ears, and mouth
Neck musculature
Chest integrity
Adequate ventilations
  Rales–rhonchi–stridor
  Wheezing–snoring
  Distant sounds
Extremities
  Grip strength
  Distal pulse
  Flexation/extension
Obvious hemorrhage
Pelvic integrity
Abdominal status
  Point–rebound–rigid
Mechanism of injury

Level of consciousness
Skin color/temperature
Vitals: B/P, P, R
Crepitus: raccoon eyes
CNS/blood: Battle's sign
Tracheal deviation
Paradoxical breathing
Heart sounds
Mini-neurological assessment
  Oriented to person, place, time
  Pupils, posture
  Level of consciousness
Capillary refill
Glasgow coma score
Ability to move
Bleeding rectally
Pulse oximetry
Bleeding vaginally
Trauma score
Burns present (see the Fire section)
Type burn

Assessment: Possible problems and other considerations:

Note: Any of the following may be a result of system insult.

Arrhythmia
Tension pneumothorax
Congenital history
Trauma (see the Auto and GSW sections)
Environmental exposure
Muffled heart tones
Cardiac disease
CVA
Pericarditis
Vaso/vagal response
Appendicitis
Ectopic pregnancy
Hepatic disease
Carcinoma

Head injury
Flail chest
Emphysema
COPD
If pregnant, fetal heart tones (see the Obstetrics section)
Respiratory disease
TIA
Pulmonary embolism
Aortic aneurysm
Pleurisy
Pancreatitis
Subarachnoid bleed
Epidural bleed

Plan: Action taken, skills performed:

Procedure		*Response*
Airway Oropharyngeal	• Time placed/who placed • Size used • Supplemental oxygen • Adjunctive equipment	• Skin color/temperature • Breath sounds • Capillary refill • Chest expansion
Esophageal	• Time placed/who placed • Supplemental oxygen • Adjunctive equipment	• Skin color/temperature • Breath sounds • Capillary refill • Chest expansion • Gastric distension
Endotracheal	• Time placed/who placed • Size used • Tube passed with cord visualization • Oral/nasal introduction	• Skin color/temperature • Breath sounds • Capillary refill • Chest expansion • Epigastric silent • Gastric distension
Suctioning	• Oral/tracheal • Time/who suctioned	• Fluid evacuated • Capillary refill • Skin color/temperature • Mental status
Cervical Spinal	• Device used Cervical collar Cervical immobilization Blanket roll KED/backboard • Time device applied • Adjunctive equipment	• Extremity pulses • Sensations • Capillary refill • Skin color/temperature • Mechanism of injury • Mini-neurological assessment: before/after
Breathing Oxygen	• Device used • Time/who applied • Liter flow • Adjunctive equipment	• Skin color/temperature • Capillary refill • Patient position • Mental status • Mucosa color
BVM/demand	• Time/who applied • Adjunctive equipment	• Skin color • Chest expansion • Gastric distension
Pulse oximetry	• Time/who applied • Type of probe	• Percent oxygen saturation

Circulation		
CPR/mechanical	• Time started	• Pulse present with compression
Monitor	• Time/who applied • Lead placed • EKG interpretation	• Skin color/temperature • Breath sounds • Before and after all treatments and medications
IV	• Time/who placed • Size of catheter • Location of IV • Fluid type	• Blood drawn • Vitals
Defib./cardio.	• Time/who placed • Watts/second used	• EKG response, before and after
External pace	• Time/who placed • Milliampere rate	• EKG response, before and after
Drug admin.	• Time/who placed • Drug type • Dosage • Route: SQ, IM, IV, ETT	• Mental status • EKG response • Vital response • Pain relief
MAST	• Time/who placed • Sections inflated • Adjunctive equipment	• Extremity pulses • Capillary refill • Mental status
Hemorrhage		
Bandage/dressing	• Time/who placed • Pressure points used • Direct pressure used • Type dressing applied • Location of splint • Adjunctive equipment	• Extremity pulses • Estimated blood loss • Capillary refill • Skin color/temperature • Sensation
Splinting	• Time/who placed • Type of splint • Location of splint • Adjunctive equipment	• Extremity pulses • Capillary refill • Distal sensation • Skin color/temperature

Obvious Death / Death Scene / Expired

Objective: Head-to-toe assessment (see "Head-to-Toe Approach"):

Cold/stiff	Rigor mortis
Pupils fixed/dilated	Lividity (livor mortis)
Medical history: chronic/acute	Advanced age
	Advanced age without history
Presenting EKG	Time element without vitals
Decapitated	Ambient air temperature
Brain matter exposed	Injury incompatible with life

Subjective: History of the patient:

General history	Mechanism of injury
Hypotension	Hypertension
All wounds noted, head to toe	Asthma
Emphysema	Diabetes
COPD	Headaches
Medications	Death in the family
Seizure activity	(see the Suicide section)

Description before death:

Pain/Type/Locations	*Precipitating events*
Sharp pain	Activity before the event
Dull pain	Activity after the event
Radiating pain	Approximate time of the incident
Crushing pain	Location of patient before
Chest–abdomen	Location of patient after
Back–head	Type of accident
Side(s)	Point of impact
Arm(s)	Patient found/position
Leg(s)	Drugs (contraband) present
Head	

A.C.B.C.

I have placed in order the way we manage a patient. It is not a list of priority, but rather a list of all skills and the considerations that one must document after treatment has taken place. It can be used in association with all three report categories or any format you choose. The left-hand column addresses the skill itself (the procedure), while the right-hand columns deal with the areas of treatment documentation and patient considerations.

Procedure	*Response*	
Airway		
Oropharyngeal	• Time placed/who placed • Size used • Supplemental oxygen • Adjunctive equipment	• Skin color/temperature • Breath sounds • Capillary refill • Chest expansion
Esophageal	• Time placed/who placed • Supplemental oxygen • Adjunctive equipment	• Skin color/temperature • Breath sounds • Capillary refill • Chest expansion • Gastric distension
Endotracheal	• Time placed/who placed • Size used • Tube passed with cord visualization • Oral/nasal introduction	• Skin color/temperature • Breath sounds • Capillary refill • Chest expansion • Epigastric silent • Gastric distension

Cricothyrotomy	• Size used • Tube passed • Chest expansion	• Breath sounds • Capillary refill
Suctioning	• Oral/tracheal • Time/who suctioned • Catheter size	• Fluid evacuated • Capillary refill • Skin color/temperature • Mental status
Cervical		
Spinal	• Device used Cervical collar Cervical immobilization Blanket roll KED/backboard • Time device applied • Adjunctive equipment	• Extremity pulses • Sensations • Capillary refill • Skin color/temperature • Mechanism of injury • Mini-neurological assessment: before/after
Breathing		
Oxygen	• Device used • Time/who applied • Liter flow • Adjunctive equipment	• Skin color/temperature • Capillary refill • Patient position • Mental status • Mucosa color
BVM/demand	• Time/who applied • Adjunctive equipment	• Skin color • Chest expansion • Gastric distension
Pulse oximetry	• Time/who applied • Type of probe	• Percent oxygen saturation
Pleural decompression	• Device used • Time/who applied • Liter flow • Adjunctive equipment	• Skin color/temperature • Capillary refill • Patient position • Mental status • Mucosa color
Circulation		
CPR/mechanical	• Time started	• Pulse present with compression
Monitor	• Time/who applied • Lead placed • EKG interpretation	• Skin color/temperature • Breath sounds • Before and after all treatments and medications
IV	• Time/who placed • Size of catheter • Location of IV • Fluid type	• Blood drawn • Vitals
Defib./cardio.	• Time/who placed • Watts/second used	• EKG response, before and after

External pace	• Time/who placed • Milliampere rate	• EKG response, before and after
Drug admin.	• Time/who placed • Drug type • Dosage • Route: SQ, IM, IV, ETT	• Mental status • EKG response • Vital response • Pain relief
MAST	• Time/who placed • Sections inflated • Adjunctive equipment	• Extremity pulses • Capillary refill • Mental status
Hemorrhage Bandage/dressing	• Time/who placed • Pressure points used • Direct pressure used • Type dressing applied • Location of splint • Adjunctive equipment	• Extremity pulses • Estimated blood loss • Capillary refill • Skin color/temperature • Sensation
Splinting	• Time/who placed device • Type of splint • Location of splint • Adjunctive equipment	• Extremity pulses • Capillary refill • Skin color/temperature • Sensation
Peritoneal Lavage	• Fluid administered • Time frame in cavity • Time/who placed	• Volume of fluid • Time started/end • Route/needle size

5

Drug Calculations

Listed here are some general guidelines to follow when handing drugs. The approach is not a teaching technique but, rather, an informative one. I have given a few drug charts that will make the calculation easier. However, because dosages vary from system to system and from region to region, check to see if these mixes match your system's protocol.

DRUG ADMINISTRATION

1. Patient's history: allergies or drug responses.
2. Validate the drug to be used *three times.*
3. Document vitals and cardiac rhythm before and after administration.
4. Document the type, amount (dose), and time the drug was administered.
5. Document the response, if any, and the time the response was noticed.

Adult Dose Rates

Bretylium Tosylate (Bretylol)

IV PUSH: Millimeters of undiluted bretylium tosylate

	Body Weight (kg)								
Dose Rate (mg/kg)	55	60	65	70	75	80	85	90	95
5	5.5	6	6.5	7	7.5	8	8.5	9	9.5
10	11	12	13	14	15	16	17	18	19
15	16.5	18	18.5	21	21.5	24	24.5	17	17.5

Drip Rate: Microdrops per minute of diluted bretylium tosylate 500 mg in 250 mL

Dose Rate (microdrops/min)	30	60	90	120
Dose Rate (mg/kg)	1	2	3	4

Dopamine Hydrochloride (Intropin)

400 mg in 250 mL = 1600 mcg/mL

	Body Weight (kg)								
Dose Rate (mcg/kg/min)	55	60	65	70	75	80	85	90	95
2.5	5	6	6	7	7	8	8	8	9
5.0	10	11	12	13	14	15	16	17	18
10.0	21	23	24	26	28	30	32	34	36
15.0	31	34	37	39	42	45	48	51	53
20.0	41	45	49	52	56	60	64	68	71
25.0	52	56	61	66	70	75	80	84	89
30.0	62	67	73	78	84	90	96	101	107
35.0	72	79	85	92	98	105	112	118	125
40.0	83	90	98	105	113	120	128	135	143
45.0	93	101	110	118	127	135	143	152	160

The result intersection of the two knowns gives the amount in mcg/min.

Epinephrine Hydrochloride (Adrenalin)

1 mg in 250 mL

Dose Rate (millidrops/min)	15	30	45	60	75	90
Dose Rate (mcg/min)	1	2	3	4	5	6

Isoproterenol (Isuprel)

2 mg in 250 mL = 4 mcg/mL

Dose Rate (mcg/min)	1	2	3	4	5	6	8	12
Concentration	15	30	45	60	75	90	120	180

The result intersection of the two knowns gives the amount in mcg/min.

Lidocaine Hydrochloride (Xylocaine)

1 g in 250 mL

Dose Rate (microdrops/min)	15	30	45	60
Dose Rate (mg)	1	2	3	4

Nipride (Sodium Nitroprusside)

50 mg in 250 mL = 200 mcg/mL

Dose Rate (mcg/kg/min)	Body Weight (kg) 55	60	65	70	75	80	85	90	95
0.5	8	9	10	11	11	12	13	14	14
1.0	17	18	20	21	23	24	26	27	29
2.0	33	36	39	42	45	48	51	54	57
3.0	50	54	59	63	68	72	77	81	86
4.0	66	72	78	84	90	96	102	108	114
5.0	83	90	98	105	113	120	128	135	143
6.0	99	108	117	126	135	144	153	162	171
7.0	116	126	137	147	158	168	179	189	200
8.0	132	144	156	168	180	192	204	216	228
9.0	149	162	176	189	203	216	230	243	257
10.0	165	180	195	210	225	240	255	270	285

The result intersection of the two knowns gives the amount in mcg/min.

Pediatric Dose Rates

	1.0 kg		2.0 kg		3.0 kg	
	Dose	Volume	Dose	Volume	Dose	Volume
NaH_2CO_3	1 mEq	1 mL	2 mEq	2 mL	3 mEq	3 mL
Epinephrine	0.01 mg	0.1 mL	0.02 mg	0.2 mL	0.03 mg	0.3 mL
Atropine	0.15 mg	1.5 mL	0.15 mg	1.5 mL	0.15 mg	1.5 mL
Lidocaine[a]	0.5 mg	0.05 mL	1.0 mg	0.1 mL	1.5 mg	0.15 mL
CaCl[b]	20.0 mg	0.2 mL	40.0 mg	0.4 mL	60.0 mg	0.6 mL
Valium[a]	0.3–0.5 mg		0.6–1.0 mg		0.9–1.5 mg	
D25%	4.0 mL		8.0 mL		12.0 mL	
Narcan	0.01 mg		0.02 mg		0.03 mg	
Lasix	1.0 mg		2.0 mg		3.0 mg	
Bretylium[b]	5.0 mg		10.0 mg		15.0 mg	

	4.0 kg		5.0 kg		6.0 kg	
NaH_2CO_3	4 mEq	4 mL	5 mEq	5 mL	6 mEq	6 mL
Epinephrine	0.04 mg	0.4 mL	0.05 mg	0.5 mL	0.06 mg	0.6 mL
Atropine	0.15 mg	1.5 mL	0.15 mg	1.5 mL	0.15 mg	1.5 mL
Lidocaine[a]	2.0 mg	0.2 mL	2.5 mg	.25 mL	3.0 mg	0.3 mL
CaCl[b]	80.0 mg	0.8 mL	100.0 mg	1.0 mL	120.0 mg	1.2 mL
Valium[a]	1.2 mg		1.5 mg		1.8 mg	
D25%	16.0 mL		20.0 mL		24.0 mL	
Narcan	0.04 mg		0.05 mg		0.06 mg	
Lasix	4.0 mg		5.0 mg		6.0 mg	
Bretylium[b]	20.0 mg		25.0 mg		30.0 mg	

	7.0 kg		8.0 kg		9.0 kg	
NaH_2CO_3	7 mEq	7 mL	8 mEq	8 mL	9 mEq	9 mL
Epinephrine	0.07 mg	0.7 mL	0.08 mg	0.8 mL	0.09 mg	0.9 mL
Atropine	0.15 mg	1.5 mL	0.16 mg	1.6 mL	0.18 mg	1.8 mL
Lidocaine[a]	3.5 mg	0.35 mL	4.0 mg	0.4 mL	4.5 mg	0.45 mL
CaCl[b]	140.0 mg	1.4 mL	160.0 mg	1.6 mL	180.0 mg	1.8 mL

Valium[a]	2.1 mg	2.4 mg	2.7 mg
D25%	28.0 mL	32.0 mL	36.0 mL
Narcan	0.07 mg	0.08 mg	0.09 mg
Lasix	7.0 mg	8.0 mg	9.0 mg
Bretylium[b]	35.0 mg	40.0 mg	45.0 mg

	10.0 kg		12.5 kg		15.0 kg	
NaH_2CO_3	10 mEq	10 mL	12.5 mEq	12.5 mL	15 mEq	15 mL
Epinephrine	0.10 mg	1.0 mL	0.125 mg	1.25 mL	0.15 mg	1.5 mL
Atropine	0.20 mg	2.0 mL	0.25 mg	2.5 mL	0.30 mg	3.0 mL
Lidocaine[a]	5.0 mg	0.5 mL	6.25 mg	0.625 mL	7.5 mg	0.75 mL
CaCl[b]	200.0 mg	2.0 mL	250.0 mg	2.5 mL	300.0 mg	3.0 mL
Valium[a]	3.0 mg		3.75 mg		4.5 mg	
D25%	40.0 mL		50.0 mL		60.0 mL	
Narcan	0.1 mg		0.125 mg		0.15 mg	
Lasix	10.0 mg		12.5 mg		15.0 mg	
Bretylium[b]	50.0 mg		62.5 mg		75.0 mg	

	17.5 kg		20.0 kg		22.5 kg	
NaH_2CO_3	17 mEq	17.5 mL	20 mEq	20.0 mL	22.5 mEq	22.5 mL
Epinephrine	0.175 mg	1.75 mL	0.2 mg	2.0 mL	0.225 mg	2.25 mL
Atropine	0.35 mg	3.5 mL	0.40 mg	4.0 mL	0.45 mg	4.5 mL
Lidocaine[a]	8.75 mg	0.875 mg	10.0 mg	1.0 mL	11.25 mg	1.125 mL
CaCl[b]	350.0 mg	3.5 mL	400.0 mg	4.0 mL	450.0 mg	4.5 mL
Valium[a]	5.25 mg		6.0 mg		6.75 mg	
D25%	70.0 mL		80.0 mL		90.0 mL	
Narcan	0.175 mg		0.20 mg		0.225 mg	
Lasix	17.5 mg		20.0 mg		22.5 mg	
Bretylium[b]	87.5 mg		100.0 mg		112.0 mg	

	25.0		30.0		35.0	
NaH_2CO_3	25 mEq	25.0 mL	30 mEq	30 mL	35 mEq	35 mL
Epinephrine	0.25 mg	2.5 mL	0.3 mg	3.0 mL	0.35 mg	3.5 mL
Atropine	0.5 mg	5.0 mL	0.5 mg	5.0 mL	0.5 mg	5.0 mL
Lidocaine[a]	12.5 mg	1.25 mL	15.0 mg	1.5 mL	17.5 mg	1.75 mL
CaCl[b]	500.0 mg	5.0 mL	500.0 mg	5.0 mL	500.0 mg	5.0 mL
Valium[a]	7.5 mg		9.0 mg		10.0 mg	
D25%	100.0 mL		120.0 mL		140.0 mL	
Narcan	0.25 mg		0.30 mg		0.35 mg	
Lasix	25.0 mg		30.0 mg		35.0 mg	
Bretylium[b]	125.0 mg		150.0 mg		175.0 mg	

[a] *Increased response.*

[b] *Contraindicated or extreme care.*

6

Commonly Misspelled Words: Medical and English

MEDICAL

Abdominal
Abdominogenital
Abduction
Aberrant
Aberration
Abortion
Abrasion
Abruptio
Abscess
Acetone
Acidosis
Acute
Adams–Stokes
Addison's Disease
Alimentary
Allergy
Alveolar
Alveoli
Alveolus
Alzheimer's
Ameba
Aminophylline
Amniocentesis
Amniotic
Ampule
Amputation
Anaphylaxis
Anatomy
Anemia
Anemic
Anesthesia
Aneurysm
Angina
Angiocardiography
Anorexia
Anoxia
Antabuse
Antecubital
Anterior
Anxiety
Aorta
Aortic
Apex
Apgar score
Apnea
Appendage
Appendectomy
Appendicitis
Appendix
Arrhythmia
Arterial
Arteriolosclerosis
Artery
Arthritis
Anthroscopy
Aseptic
Aspect
Asphyxia
Aspirate
Aspiration
Aspirin
Asthma
Asthmatic
Asymmetry
Atopic
Atrial
Atrium
Atropine
Auscultation
Autonomic
Avulsion

Babinski's reflex
Bandage
Basal
Benign
Bends
Bigeminal
Bigeminy
Bilateral
Biot's breathing

Blood
Bolus
Brachial
Bradycardia
Bradypnea
Bradyrhythmia
Breech
Bronchial
Bruise
Bundle branch block

Cancer
Cannula
Capillary
Carcinogenic
Cardiac
Cardiomyoliposis
Cardionecrosis
Cardiopericarditis
Cardiovascular
Cardioversion
Carotid
Catheter
Catheterization
Cerebrospinal
Cervical
Cesarean section
Chest
Cheyne–Stokes
Cholesterol
Chronic
Circulatory
Circumcision
Cirrhosis
Clavicle
Clavicular
Cocaine
Coccygeal
Codeine
Conception
Conceptus
Concussion
Condensation
Congestion
Congestive
Conjunct
Conjunctivitis
Conscious
Consciousness
Constipation
Constriction
Contraction
Contraindication
Contrecoup

Corneal
Coronary
Cough
Cramp
Cranium
Crepitus
Cyanosis
Cyanotic

Decapitation
Decerebrate
Decubitus
Defecation
Defibrillation
Deformity
Dehydration
Delirium Tremens
Deltoid
Deviation
Dextrose
Diabetes
Diagnosis
Dialysis
Diaphoretic
Diaphragmatic
Diarrhea
Diastolic
Dilatation
Disease
Dissociation
Diverticulitis
Duodenum
Dyslexia
Dysphasia
Dyspnea
Dyspneic

Ecchymosis
Eclampsia
Ectopic
Edema
Embolism
Embryo
Embryonic
Emesis
Emphysema
Encephalitis
Endoscopy
Epiglottitis
Epilepsy
Epistaxis
Evisceration
Expiration
Extrasystole

Febrile
Fibula
Fistula
Fontanelle

Gangrane
Gastric
Genitalia
Gestation
Glaucoma
Glottis

Hematemesis
Hematoma
Hemihypesthesia
Hemiparaplegia
Hemophilia
Hemorrhage
Hernia
Hyperpnea
Hyperthyroid
Hypertrophy
Hypoglycemia
Hypoglycemic
Hysterectomy

Idioventricular
Ileac
Ileocolitis
Immune
Immunity
Immunization
Impaction
Incontinence
Indigestion
Infarct
Infraction
Infection
Infectious
Inflammation
Influenza
Infusion
Ingestion
Injection
Injury
Insomnia
Inspiration
Inspiratory
Insufficiency
Insulin
Intensity
Interferon
Intestinal
Intoxication

Intracranial
Intramuscular
Intraosseous
Intubate
Intubation
Ipecac
Ischium

Jaundice
Joule
Jugular

Kidney

Laceration
Laryngeal
Larynx
Laxative
Lethal
Lethargic
Leukemia
Ligament
Livedo
Lividity
Lumbar

Malformation
Malignant
Malleolus
Mandible
Marijuana
Maxilla
Measles
Meconium
Mediastinal
Medication
Meningitis
Menopause
Menstrual cycle
Menstruation
Miscarriage
Mitral
Morbidity
Morphine
Mortality
Mucosa
Mucus
Murmur
Muscular
Musculature

Narcotic
Nasal
Nausea
Nebulizer
Neonatal
Nephritis
Nitroglycerin
Nitrous Oxide
Nocturnal

Obstetrical
Occult
Odor
Oligopnea
Orthopedic
Ovarian
Ovulation
Oxygen
Oxygenate
Oxygenation

Palpation
Pancarditis
Pancreas
Pancreatitis
Paralysis
Paraplegia
Paraplegic
Parenteral
Parkinson
Paroxysmal
Patency
Patent
Pediatrician
Pediatrics
Penis
Perfusion
Pericarditis
Perineum
Peritoneum
Phalanges
Pharyngeal
Pharynx
Phlebitis
Photosensitivity
Physician
Physiological
Placenta
Pleurisy
Pneumonia
Pneumothorax
Posterior
Postictal
Preeclampsia
Pregnancy
Pregnant (gravid)
Prescription
Productive
Projection
Prolapse
Prone
Prostate
Psychiatry
Psychologist
Pupillary

Quadrant
Quadriplegia

Rales
Rectal
Respiration
Resuscitator
Retrograde
Rheumatic
Rigidity
Rigor Mortis
Rubella

Sacral
Sacrum
Saliva
Scapula
Scapular
Scrotum
Secretion
Sedation
Sedative
Seizure
Sepsis
Septic
Skull
Sputum
Sternum
Stoma
Stridor
Sublingual
Superior
Supine
Syncope
Syringe

Tachycardia
Tamponade
Tetanus
Thoracic
Thorax
Thyroid
Tonsillitis
Toxemia
Trechea
Trendelenburg
Triage
Tuberculosis
Turgor

Ulcer
Umbilical
Umbilicus
Unconsciousness
Urinate
Uterine

Vaccination
Vagina
Valsalva
Ventilation
Vertigo
Viscera
Voluntary
Vomiting

Wound

Xiphoid

Yeast

Zoster

ENGLISH

Abandon
Abbreviate
Ability
Abnormal
Aboard
About
Abroad
Abrupt
Absent
Absolute
Absorb
Abuse
Abusive
Accelerator
Access
Accessory
Accident
Accommodate
Accompany
Accomplish
Achieve
Acknowledge
Activity
Actual
Acute
Adequate
Adjacent
Adjunct
Administer
Alkali
Alleviate
Alternate
Ambiguous
Anxiety
Appropriate

Bacteria
Bandage
Battalion
Belligerent
Boisterous
Brine
Bureau

Campaign
Challenge
Chlorine
Cigarette
Circumstance
Clandestine
Compartment
Considerable
Consistent
Constituent
Consultant
Contagious
Contaminate
Contingency
Correlate

Degenerate
Demeanor
Diagnosis
Difficult

Either
Electricity
Electrocute
Essential
Evidence
Extinguish

Fatigue
Flaccid
Frequent

Grimace

Hemorrhage

Illiterate
Incident
Incipient
Individual
Infiltrate
Integrity
Itch

Judge

Kindergarten

Lieutenant

Malnutrition
Marble
Maximum
Mechanism
Memorandum
Mosquito

Necessary
Nervous

Observe
Occasional
Ointment
Oval

Paralysis
Peculiar
Perforate
Proximity

Quality

Receive
Relapse
Relief
Relieve

Sensation
Simultaneous
Situation
Spontaneous
Supplement
Susceptible

Tangible
Technician

Usual

Vaccination
Variety
Vicinity
Violent

A

Medical Abbreviations

Abbreviation	Meaning
a	Before
A/A, Auto	Auto accident
Abd	Abdomen
AC	Antecubital
ALS	Advanced life support
A/O × 3	Alert and oriented to person, place, and time
A/P	Anterior/posterior, looking anteriorly toward the posterior
ASA	Aspirin
Bicarb	Sodium bicarbonate
b.i.d.	Twice a day
BLS	Basic life support
BM	Bowel movement
BP, B/P	Blood pressure
B/S	Breath sounds
B.S.	Bowel sounds
BSA	Body surface area
BVM	Bag valve mask
c̄	With
CAD	Coronary artery disease
C/C	Chief complaint
CA	Cancer
cc	Cubic centimeter

cc/hr	Cubic centimeter per hour
cc/min	Cubic centimeter per minute
CCU	Coronary Care Unit
CHF	Congestive Heart Failure
CID	Cervical Immobilization Device
CNS	Central Nervous System
COPD	Chronic Obstructive Pulmonary Disease
CPR	Cardiopulmonary resuscition
CSF	Cerebrospinal fluid
C-spine	Cervical spine
CVA	Cerebrovascular accident
D_5W	5% Dextrose in water
D/C	Discontinue
Defib	Defibrillated
Dr	Doctor
DT's	Delirium tremens
Dx	Diagnosis
ECG, EKG	Electrocardiogram
Elix, el	Elixir
EMD	Electromechanical dissociation
EOA	Esophageal obdurator airway
Epi	Epinephrine
Est	Estimated
ETA	Estimated time of arrival
ETD	Estimated time of departure
EtOH	Ethyl alcohol
ETT, E/TT, ET	Endotracheal tube
Et	And
Exp	Expiratory
Ex	From
Fld., fl	Fluid
FOB	Foreign object/body
Fx	Fracture
G	Gravida
GCS	Glasgow coma score
GI	Gastrointestinal tract
gm	Gram
gm/hr	Grams per hour
gm/min	Grams per minute
GSW	Gunshot wound
gtt	Drops
gtt/hr	Drops per hour
gtt/min	Drops per minute
h	Hour
Hx	History
IM	Intramuscular

Inf	Infusion
Insp	Inspiratory
IV	Intravenous
IVP	IV push
IVR	Idioventricular rhythm
JVD	Jugular vein distention
Kg	Kilograms
KVO, TKO	Keep vein open, to keep open
L	Liter
Ⓛ	Left
L-II	Lead 2
Lb	Pound
LBB	Long backboard
LLQ	Left lower quadrant
LOC	Level of consciousness
L-spine	Lumbar spine
LUQ	Left upper quadrant
L/min	Liters per minute
L/R, LR, RL	Lactated Ringer's
M	Meter
MAE	Moves all extremities
mcg	Microgram
mc/gtt	Microdrops
mcg/hr	Micrograms per hour
mcg/min	Micrograms per minute
Med	Medications
mEq	Milliquivalent
mg	Milligram
mg/hr	Milligram per hour
mg/min	Milligram per minute
min	Minutes
MAST	Military antishock trousers; medical antishock trousers
NC, N/C	Nasal cannula
Neg	Negative
NKA	No known allergies
No.	Number
Non rep.	Don't repeat
Noxt.	At night
NPO	Nothing by mouth
NROM	Normal range of motion
NV, N/V	Nausea and vomiting
NS, N/S	Normal saline
NSR	Normal sinus rhythm
Nitro	Nitroglycerin
Occ	Occasional

OD	Overdose
o.d.	Right eye
o.l.	Left eye
Omn. hor.	Every hour
OPA	Oralpharyngeal airway
O_2	Oxygen
O.S.	Left eye
O.U.	Both eyes
p	After
P	Pulse
P/A	Posteriorly toward anterior
p. ae.	Equal parts
pil	Pills
PE	Pulmonary edema
Palp, Pal,	Palpitation
Ped, Peds	Pediatrics
PEARL	Pupils equal and reactive to light
po	By mouth
prn	As needed
Pt	Patient
PVC	Premature ventricular contraction
Q.h.	Every hour
Q.2h.	Every two hours
Q.3h.	Every three hours
q	Each, every
q.i.d.	Four times daily
Ⓡ	Right
R	Respirations
RLQ	Right lower quadrant
R/O, RO	Rule out
ROM	Range of motion
RUQ	Right upper quadrant
s	Without
SL, Sub/ling	Sublingual
SOB	Short of breath
S-spine	Sacral spine
STAT	Immediately
SVT	Supraventricular tachycardia
syr.	Syrup
T	Temperature
tab.	Tablet
TIA	Transient ischemic attack
t.i.d.	Three times daily
t.i.n.	Three times nightly
TKO	To keep open
T-spine	Thoracic spine

Tx	Treatment
TOT	Turned over to
Uncon	Unconscious
UTI	Urinary tract infection
VD	Venereal disease
VF	Ventricular fibrillation
Vol	Volume
VT	Ventricular tachycardia
VS, V/S	Vital signs
WS, W/S	Watt-seconds
Wt	Weight
Y/O	Years old

B

Patient Scoring

THE APGAR SCORING METHOD

Sign	0	1	2	Score 1 min	Score 5 min
Heart rate	Absent	Below 100	Over 100		
Respiration (effort)	Absent	Slow and irregular	Normal; crying		
Muscle tone	Limp	Some flexion—extremities	Active; good motion in extremities		
Irritability	No response	Crying; some motion	Crying; vigorous		
Skin color	Bluish or paleness	Pink or typical newborn color; hands and feet are blue	Pink or typical newborn color; entire body		
			TOTAL SCORE		

Source: Harvey D. Grant, et al., Brady Emergency Care, *5th ed., (Englewood Cliffs, NJ: Prentice Hall, 1990) p. 444.*

THE CHAMPION SACCO TRAUMA SCORE

The Trauma Score is used to give each injured patient a numerical score that can be used to estimate the severity of injury. The patient is graded in terms of cardiopulmonary and neurologic functions. Each category receives a numerical score. A high number indicates normal function, while a low number signifies impaired function. The numbers are totaled to give a Trauma Score. The lowest possible score is 1 (severe impairment). The highest possible score is 16 (normal for all categories).

The use of the Trauma Score can help to determine the order of care and transport, the level of care required, and if transport to a special facility is needed.

Each patient should be scored during the initial assessment and each time that vital signs are taken.

The following is based on the Trauma Score developed by Champion and Sacco. For additional information, see: Champion HR, Sacco WJ, Carnazzo AJ, et al: Trauma Score. *Critical Care Medicine* 9 (9): 672-676, 1981. Note that variations of this procedure have been adopted by some EMS Systems.

WARNING: Follow local guidelines if you are allowed to apply painful stimuli to a patient. Your local protocol should include what actions you may take when the mechanism of injury or state of consciousness indicates possible spinal injury.

TRAUMA SCORE

Respiratory Rate	10-24/min	4	
	24-35/min	3	
	36/min or greater	2	
	1-9/min	1	
	None	0	
Respiratory Expansion	Normal	1	
	Retractive	0	
Systolic Blood Pressure	90 mmHg or greater	4	
	70-89 mmHg	3	
	50-69 mmHg	2	
	0-49 mmHg	1	
	No Pulse	0	
Capillary Refill	Normal	2	
	Delayed	1	
	None	0	
Cardiopulmonary Assessment			

GLASGOW COMA SCALE

Eye Opening	Spontaneous	4	
	To Voice	3	
	To Pain	2	
	None	1	
Verbal Response	Oriented	5	
	Confused	4	
	Inappropriate Words	3	
	Incomprehensible Words	2	
	None	1	
Motor Response	Obeys Command	6	
	Localizes Pain	5	
	Withdraw (pain)	4	
	Flexion (pain)	3	
	Extension (pain)	2	
	None	1	
Glasgow Coma Score Total			

TOTAL GLASGOW COMA SCALE POINTS

14 – 15 = 5	
11 – 13 = 4	
8 – 10 = 3	
5 – 7 = 2	
3 – 4 = 1	

CONVERSION = APPROXIMATELY ONE-THIRD TOTAL VALUE

Neurologic Assessment	

Total Trauma Score = Cardiopulmonary + Neurologic	

Source: Harvey D. Grant, et al., Brady Emergency Care, *5th edition, (Englewood Cliffs, NJ: Prentice Hall, 1990) pp. 78 and 79.*

TRAUMA SCORE CONTINUED

SCORING THE PATIENT

There are four elements to the cardiopulmonary assessment. The numerical values are added together to produce a cardiopulmonary score.

There are three elements to the neurological assessment. These are derived from the Glasgow Coma Score. Each category of the Glasgow Coma Score is given a numerical value. These numerical values are added together to produce a subtotal. This number is then reduced by approximately one-third its value to produce the neurologic assessment score.

The cardiopulmonary assessment and the neurologic assessment scores are added together to give the Trauma Score.

For example, a patient has a respiratory rate of 30 breaths per minute (3), retractive chest movements (0), a systolic blood pressure of 80 mmHg (3), and delayed capillary refill (1). The total score for cardiopulmonary function is 3+0+3+1=7.

This same patient shows no eye opening (1), no verbal response (1), and an extension reaction to pain (2). Added together, the total is 4. Approximately one-third of this number is 1. The cardiopulmonary and neurologic scores are added together (7+1) to give a Trauma Score of 8.

TRAUMA SCORE DEFINITIONS

RESPIRATION RATE

The number of respirations (1 inspiration and 1 expiration) in 30 seconds, multiplied by two.

RESPIRATION EXPANSION

NORMAL – clearly visible chest wall movements that are associated with breathing.

RETRACTIVE – the use of accessory muscles (neck and abdominal muscles) to assist with breathing.

SYSTOLIC BLOOD PRESSURE

The systolic pressure recorded by auscultation or palpation (see pages 60-61).

CAPILLARY REFILL

This is determined by pressing a nail bed, the skin on the forehead, or the lining of the mouth (oral mucosa) until there is a loss of normal color (blanching or turning white). The pressure is released and the time for color return is measured. Normal return of color will take place in approximately two seconds (about the time it takes to say to yourself, "capillary refill").

NORMAL REFILL – the color returns within two seconds.

DELAYED REFILL – the color returns sometime after two seconds.

NONE – there is no indication of capillary refill.

GLASGOW COMA SCALE DEFINITIONS

EYE OPENING

This test is valid only if there is no injury or swelling that prevents the patient from opening the eyes.

SPONTANEOUS – the patient opens his or her eyes without any stimulation.

TO VOICE – the patient will open his or her eyes in response to your request. Say, "Open your eyes." If the patient's eyes remain unopened, shout the command.

TO PAIN – if the patient does not open his or her eyes in response to your voice command, pinch the back of his or her hand or the skin at the ankles (apply the stimulus to an uninjured limb).

VERBAL RESPONSE

ORIENTED – an aroused patient should be able to tell you his or her name, where he or she is, and the date in terms of the year and month.

CONFUSED – the patient cannot give accurate responses, but he or she is able to say phrases or sentences and perhaps take part in a conversation.

INAPPROPRIATE WORDS – the patient says one or several inappropriate words, usually in response to a physical stimulus. Often, the patient will curse or call for a specific person. This may happen without any stimulus.

INCOMPREHENSIBLE SOUNDS – the patient mumbles, groans, or moans in response to stimuli.

NO VERBAL RESPONSE – repeated stimulation will not cause the patient to make any sounds.

MOTOR RESPONSE

OBEYS COMMANDS – this is limited by the apparent nature of the patient's injuries and the injuries that can be associated with the mechanism of injury. The patient is asked to perform a simple task such as moving a specific finger or holding up two fingers.

If the patient does not carry out the command, painful stimuli can be utilized by applying firm pressure to an uninjured nail bed for five seconds or pinching the skin on the back of an uninjured hand or at an uninjured ankle.

LOCALIZES PAIN – the patient reaches to the source of the pain. Often, the patient will try to remove your hand from the pain site.

WITHDRAWS – the patient moves the limb rapidly away from the source of the pain. The arm may be moved away from the trunk.

FLEXION – the patient slowly bends the joint (elbow or knee) in an attempt to move away from the pain. The forearm and hand may be held against the trunk.

EXTENSION – the patient will straighten a limb in an effort to escape the pain. The movement appears slow and "stiff." There may be an internal rotation of the shoulder and forearm.

NONE – the patient does not respond to the repeated application of the stimulus.

NOTE: A special thanks is given to the people at Emergency Health Services, Department of Health, Commonwealth of Pennsylvania for their help in supplying information for this figure.

C

Anatomy and Physiological Charts

Membranes

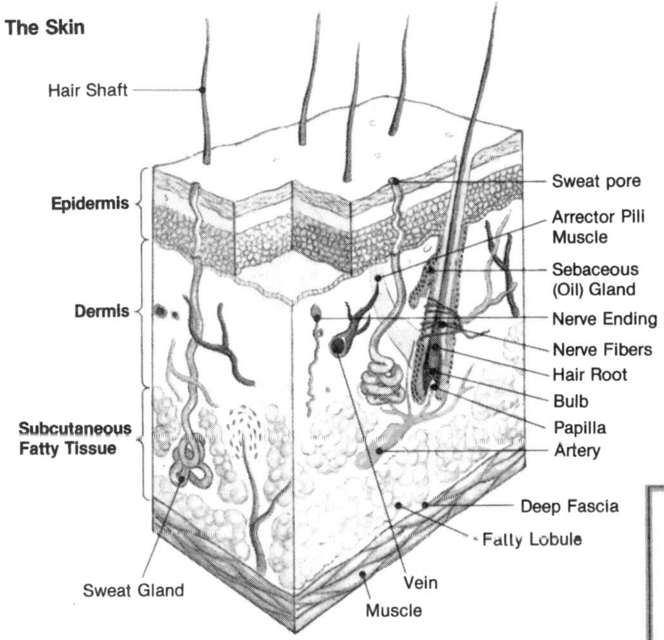

The skin is the largest organ of the body. In the adult the skin covers about 3000 square inches (1.75 square meters) and weighs about 6 pounds. It is involved with protection, insulation, thermal regulation, excretion, and the production of vitamin D.

Membranes

Membranes cover or line body structures to provide protection from injury and infection. There are four major classes of membranes. Mucous membranes line those structures that open to the outside world (for example, the mouth, the airway, digestive tract, urinary tract, and vagina). Serous membranes line the closed body cavities and cover the outsides of organs. The cutaneous membrane is the skin. Synovial membranes line joints to reduce friction during movement.

A serous membrane that covers an organ is called a visceral layer. The term parietal layer is used for the part of the serous membrane that lines a cavity. The serous membrane in the thoracic cavity is called pleura (for example, the parietal pleura lines the chest cavity). In the abdominal cavity, it is called peritoneum (for example, the parietal peritoneum). A double layer of peritoneum is called mesentery. The membrane that lines the sac surrounding the heart is pericardium.

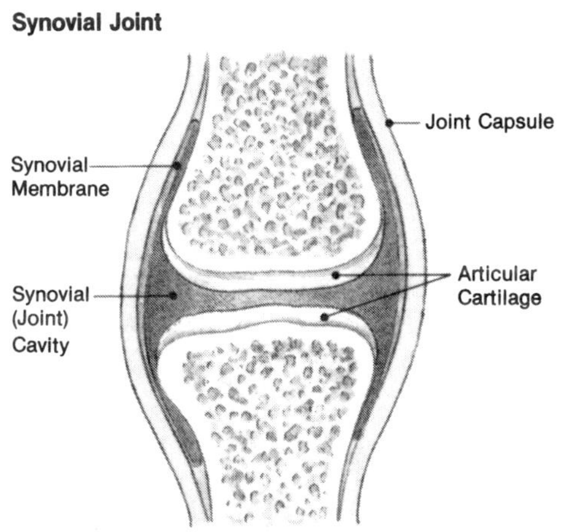

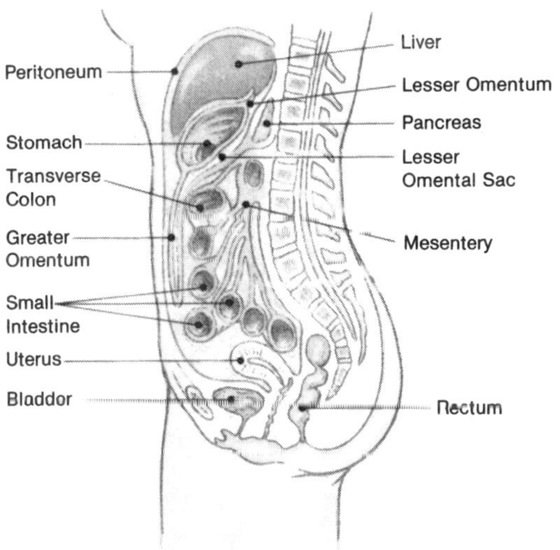

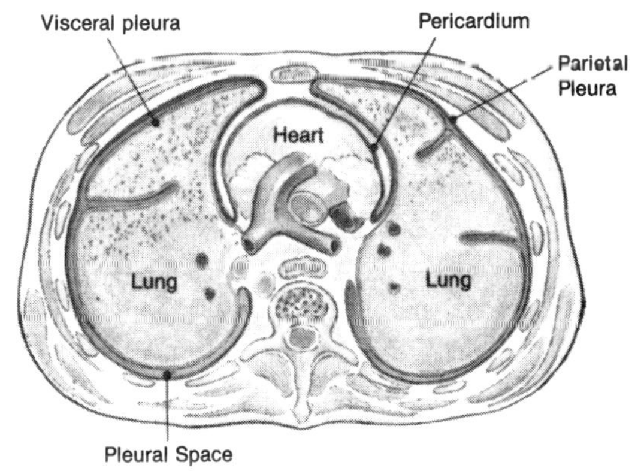

SOURCE: *Harvey D. Grant, et al.,* Brady Emergency Care, *5th edition, (Englewood Cliffs, NJ: Prentice Hall, 1990) p. 45.*

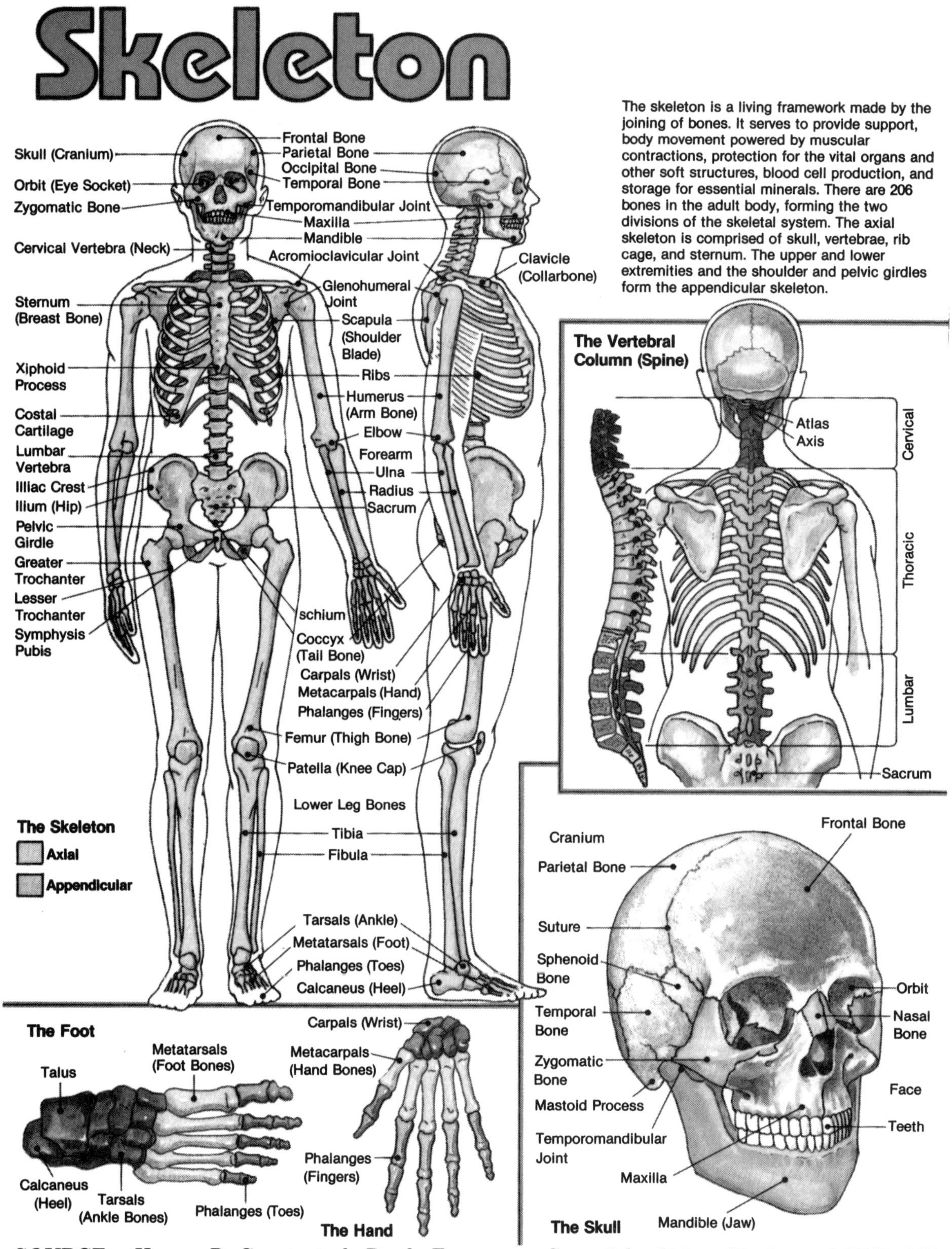

SOURCE: Harvey D. Grant, et al., Brady Emergency Care, *5th edition, (Englewood Cliffs, NJ: Prentice Hall, 1990) p. 46.*

Muscles

The Muscular System

The tissues of the muscular system comprise 40 to 50% of the body's weight. The skeletal muscles of the body are voluntary muscles, subject to conscious control. They exhibit the properties of excitability; that is, they will react to nerve stimulus. Once stimulated, skeleton muscles are quick to contract and can relax and very quickly be ready for another contraction. There are 501 separate skeletal muscles that provide contractions for movement, coordinated support for posture, and heat production. Muscles connect to bones by way of tendons.

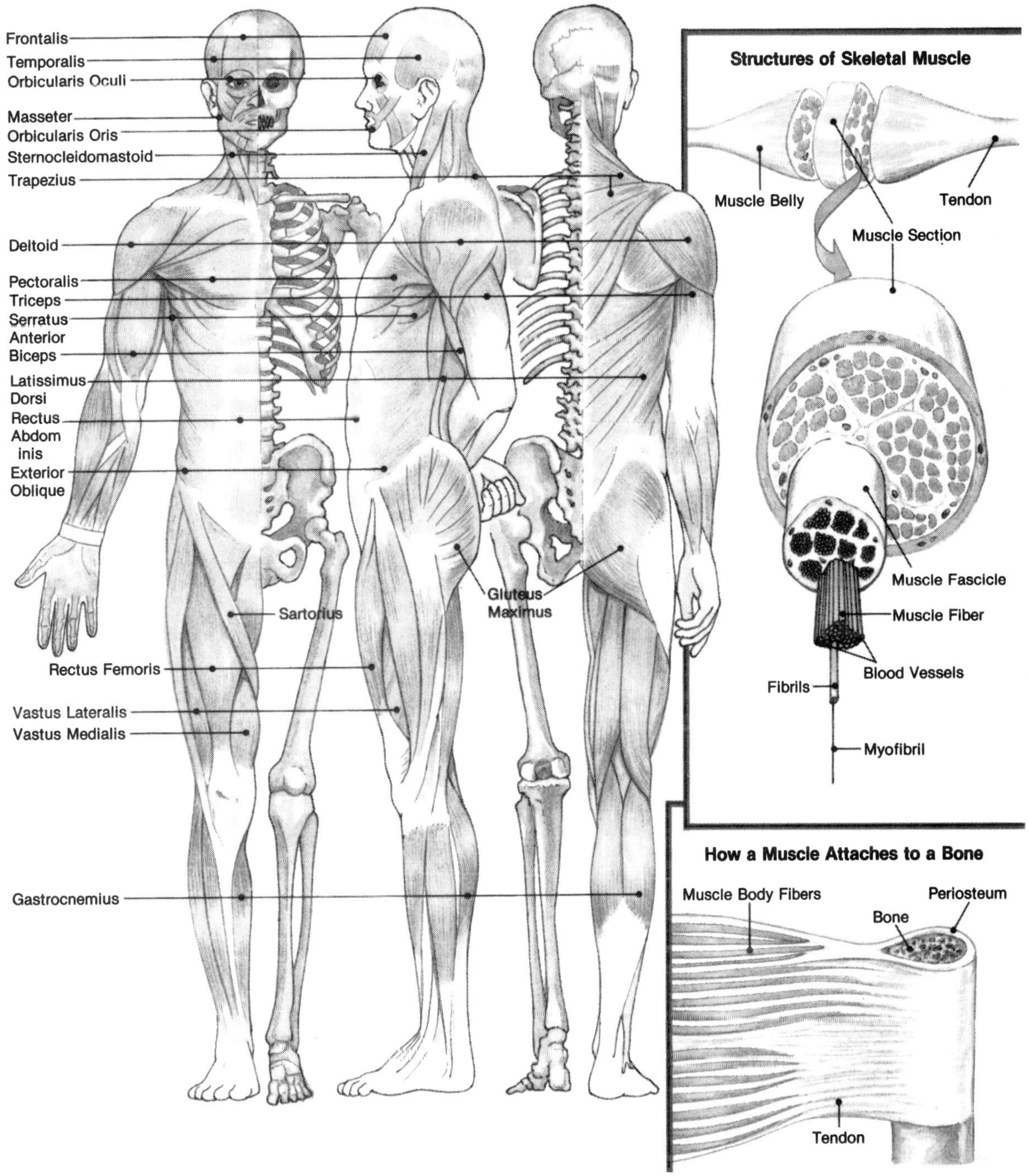

SOURCE: *Harvey D. Grant, et al.,* Brady Emergency Care, *5th edition, (Englewood Cliffs, NJ: Prentice Hall, 1990) p. 47.*

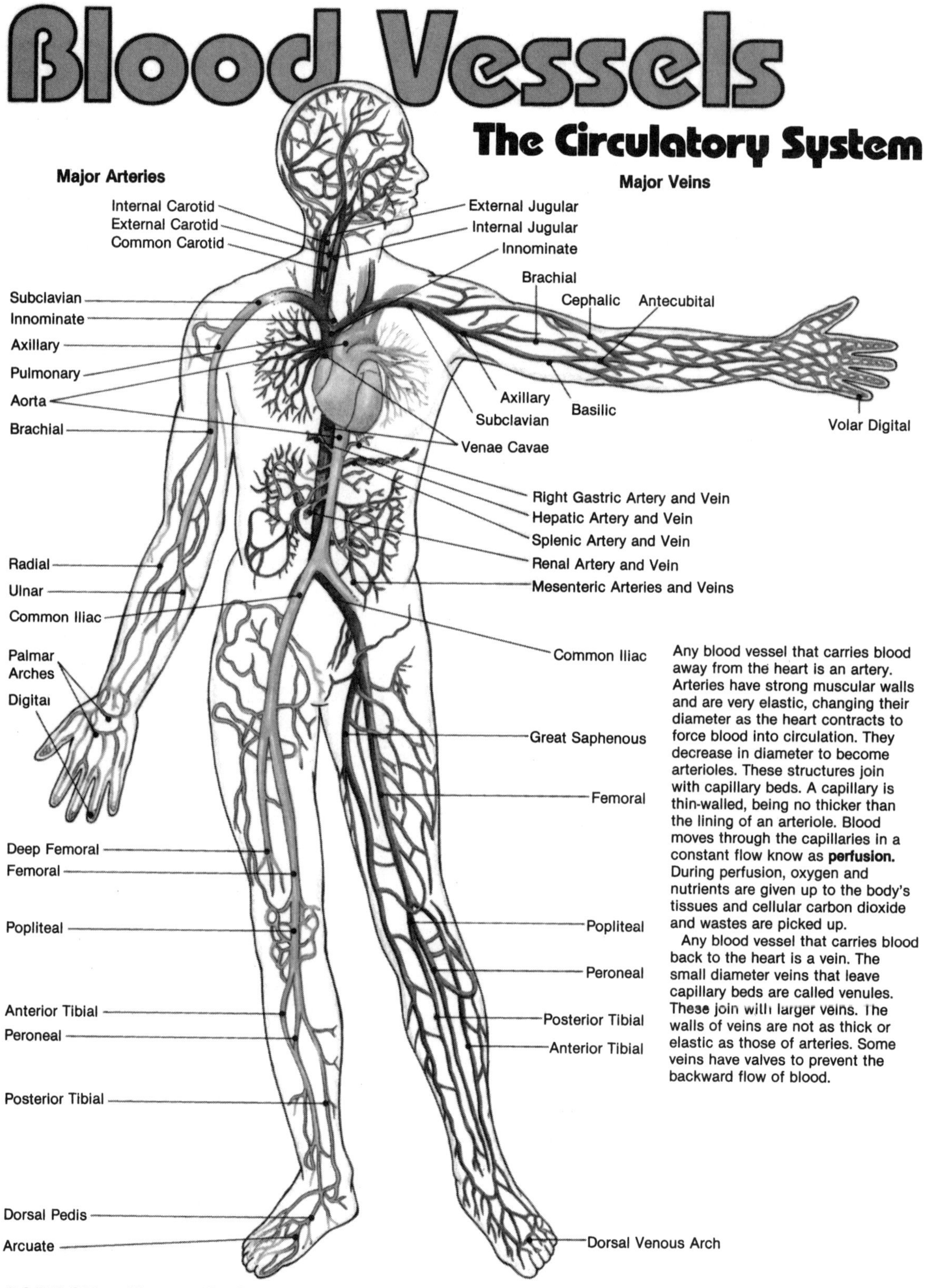

Any blood vessel that carries blood away from the heart is an artery. Arteries have strong muscular walls and are very elastic, changing their diameter as the heart contracts to force blood into circulation. They decrease in diameter to become arterioles. These structures join with capillary beds. A capillary is thin-walled, being no thicker than the lining of an arteriole. Blood moves through the capillaries in a constant flow know as **perfusion.** During perfusion, oxygen and nutrients are given up to the body's tissues and cellular carbon dioxide and wastes are picked up.

Any blood vessel that carries blood back to the heart is a vein. The small diameter veins that leave capillary beds are called venules. These join with larger veins. The walls of veins are not as thick or elastic as those of arteries. Some veins have valves to prevent the backward flow of blood.

SOURCE: Harvey D. Grant, et al., Brady Emergency Care, *5th edition, (Englewood Cliffs, NJ: Prentice Hall, 1990) p. 49.*

Nervous System

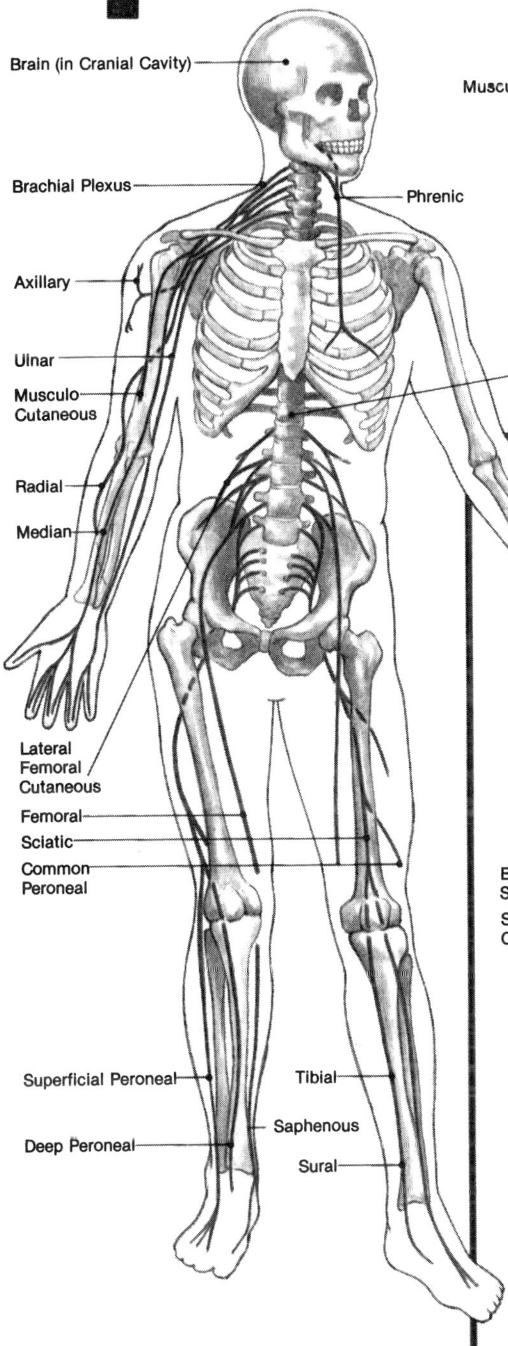

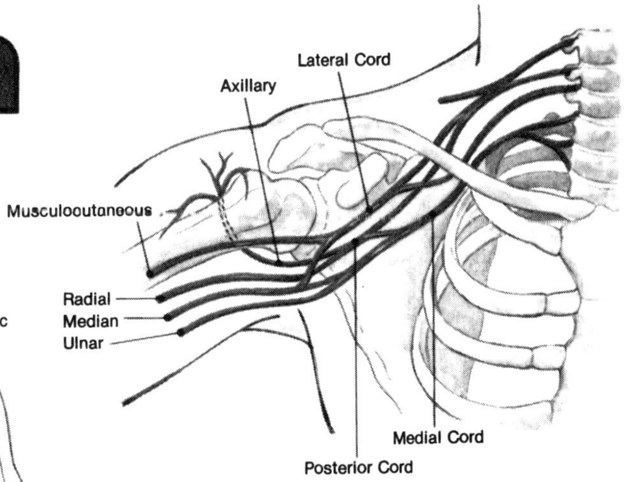

Major Nerves of the Shoulder

Autonomic Nervous System

The autonomic nervous system affects the heart, blood vessels, digestive tract, salivary and digestive glands, pancreas, liver, spleen, anal sphincter, kidneys, urinary bladder, urinary sphincter, adrenal glands, thyroid gland, gonads, genitalia, nasal lining, larynx, bronchi, lungs, iris and ciliary muscles of the eyes, tear glands, and hair muscles. Impulses can increase or slow heart rate, stimulate dilation or constriction of blood vessels, cause glands to secrete or decrease secretion, initiate or inhibit contractions in the bladder, stimulate or decrease a wave of muscle contraction along the digestive tract, and many other essential body activities.

Sympathetic (partial representation) **Parasympathetic**

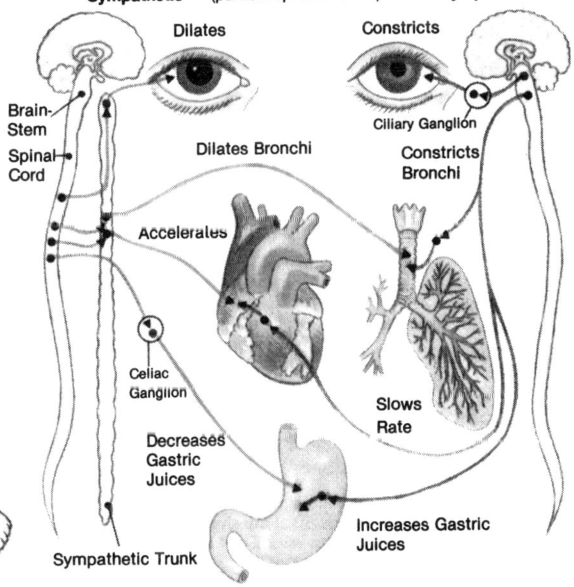

SOURCE: Harvey D. Grant, et al., **Brady Emergency Care,** *5th edition, (Englewood Cliffs, NJ: Prentice Hall, 1990) p. 51.*

Respiration

The Respiratory System

The airway consists of structures involved with the conduction and exchange of air. Conduction is the movement of air to and from the exchange levels of the lungs. Air enters through the nose (primary) and mouth (secondary) and travels down the pharynx to enter the larynx. After passing through the larynx, air enters the trachea. At its distal end, the trachea branches into the right and left primary bronchi. These bronchi branch into secondary bronchi, which then branch into the bronchioles. Some of the bronchioles end as closed tubes. Air movement in them helps the lungs expand. The rest of the bronchioles carry the air to the exchange levels of the lungs.

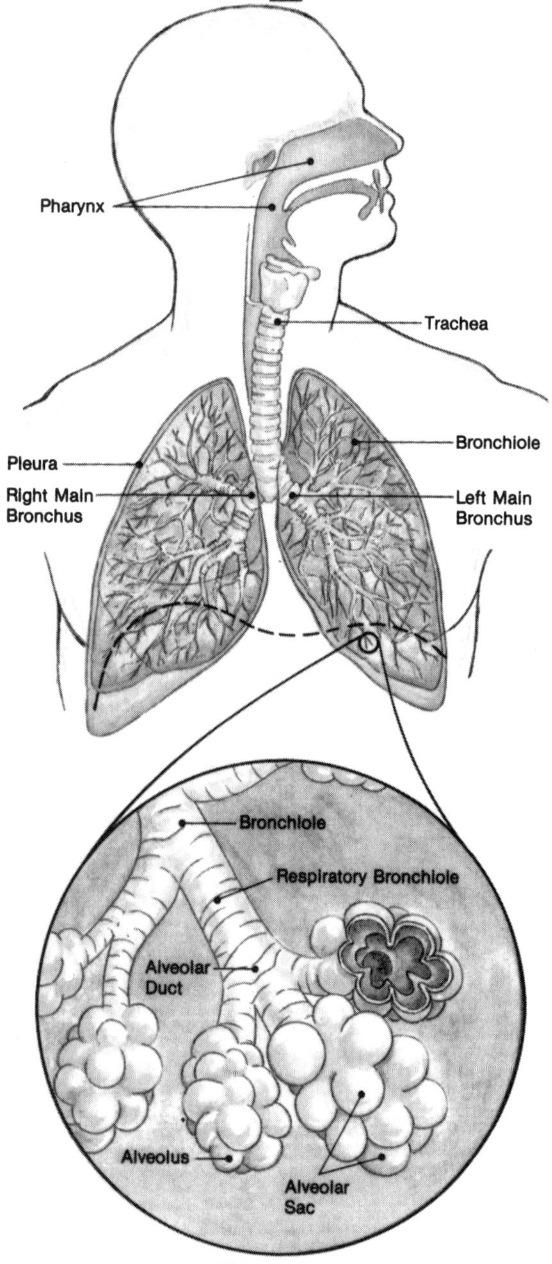

Alveolar Sacs

The respiratory bronchioles turn into alveolar ducts. These form alveolar sacs that are made up of the alveoli. Gas exchange takes place between the alveoli and the capillaries in the lungs.

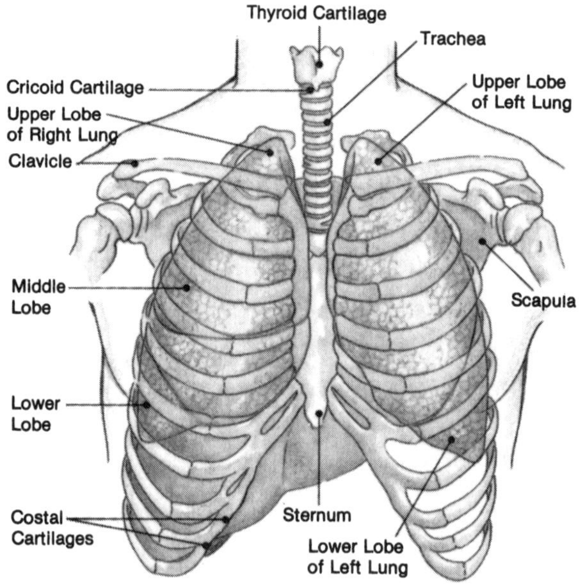

Exchange at the Alveolus

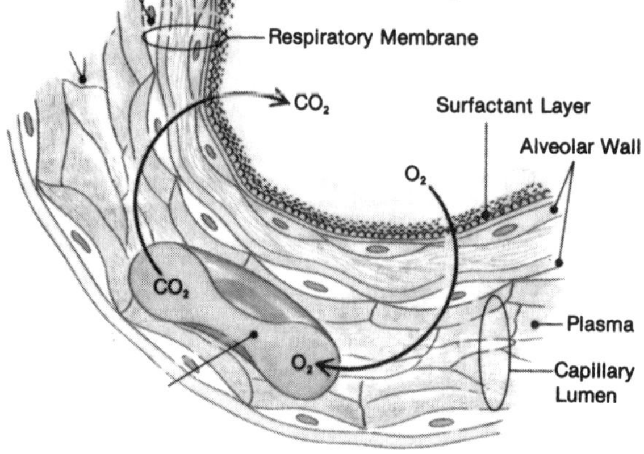

SOURCE: Harvey D. Grant, et al., Brady Emergency Care, *5th edition, (Englewood Cliffs, NJ: Prentice Hall, 1990) p. 52.*

Digestion

The Digestive System

The digestive system includes the digestive tract and various supportive structures and accessory glands. The tract begins at the oral cavity with the teeth and tongue. The salivary glands release saliva into the mouth to moisten food for swallowing. The tract continues down the throat to the esophagus, through the cardiac sphincter, and into the stomach. Acid and digestive enzymes are added to the food to produce chyme. The chyme passes through the pyloric sphincter to enter the small intestine. Digestive enzymes from the pancreas and bile from the liver are added to the chyme. The process of digestion and absorption are completed in the small intestine. Wastes are carried through the ileocecal valve into the large intestine. The wastes are moved to the rectum, from where they can be expelled through the anus.

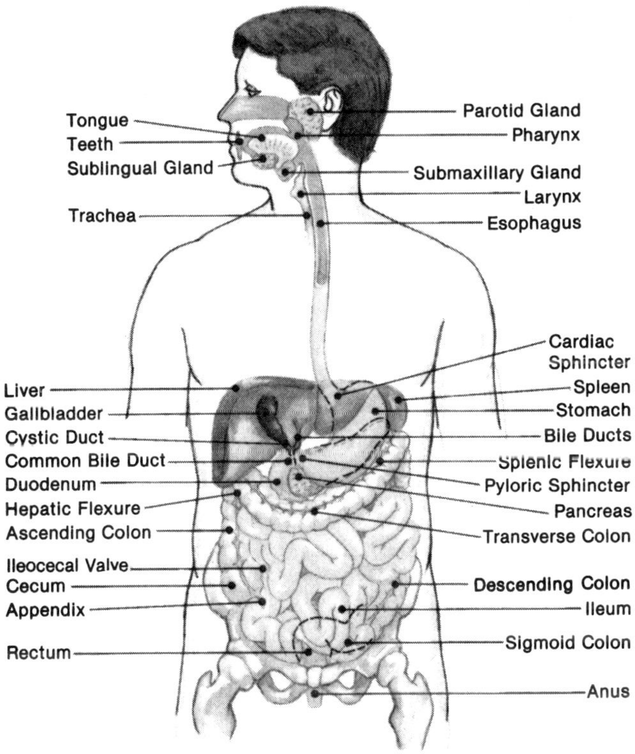

Organs of the Digestive System

Liver, Stomach, and Pancreas

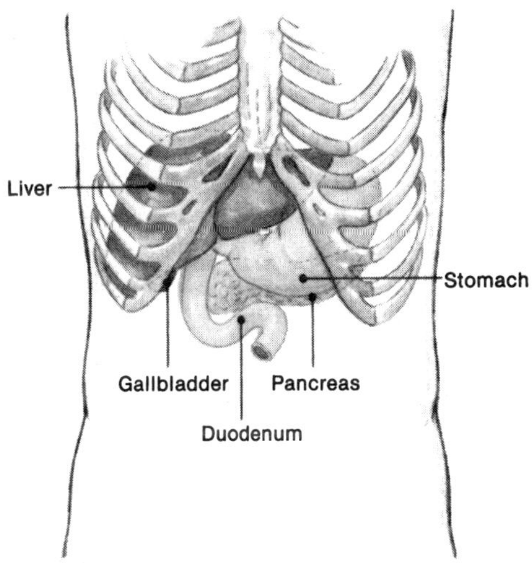

Large Intestine

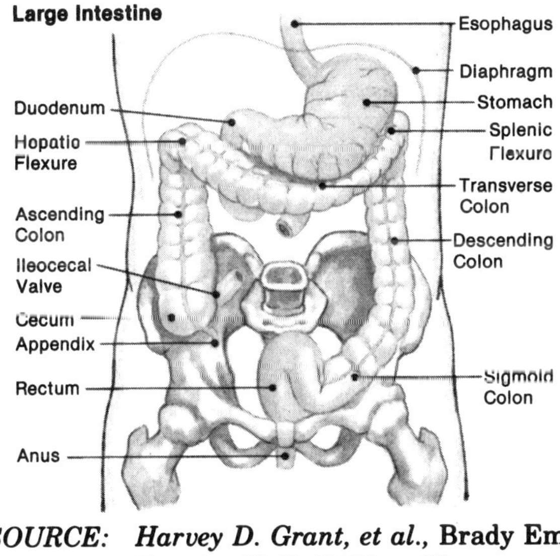

Small Intestine

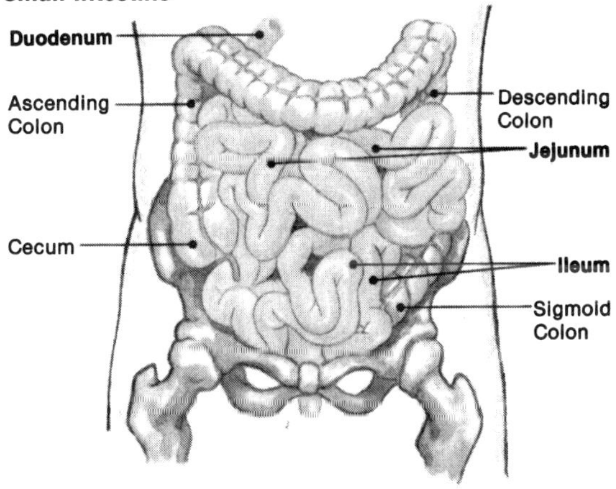

SOURCE: Harvey D. Grant, et al., Brady Emergency Care, *5th edition, (Englewood Cliffs, NJ: Prentice Hall, 1990) p. 53.*

Excretion The Urinary System

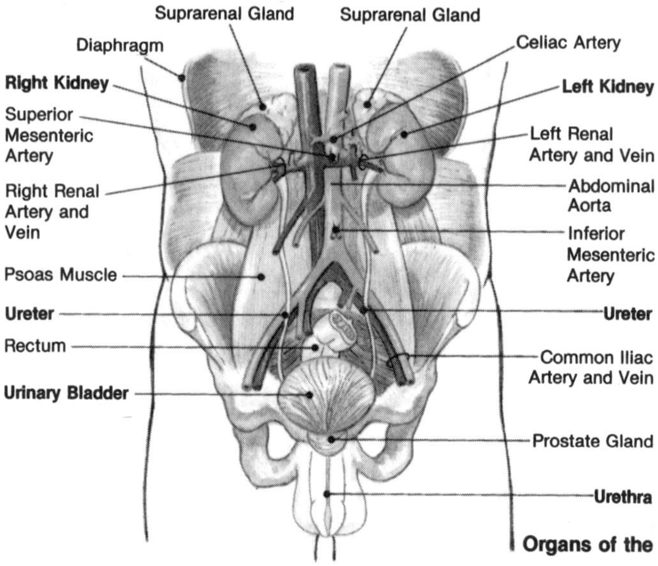

Organs of the Urinary System

The urinary system is part of the body's excretory structures (urinary system, lungs, sweat glands, and intestine). The kidneys remove the wastes of chemical activities (metabolism) in the body. These wastes are removed from the blood to produce urine. At the same time, the kidneys remove certain excess compounds, regulate the blood pH (acid-base balance), and the concentration of sodium, potassium, chlorine, glucose and other important chemicals.

The Nephron

Each kidney is made up of microscopic nephrons. Both wastes and needed chemicals are filtered from the blood. As these materials are passed through the nephron, the needed compounds (including water) are sent back into the blood. Wastes are collected as urine.

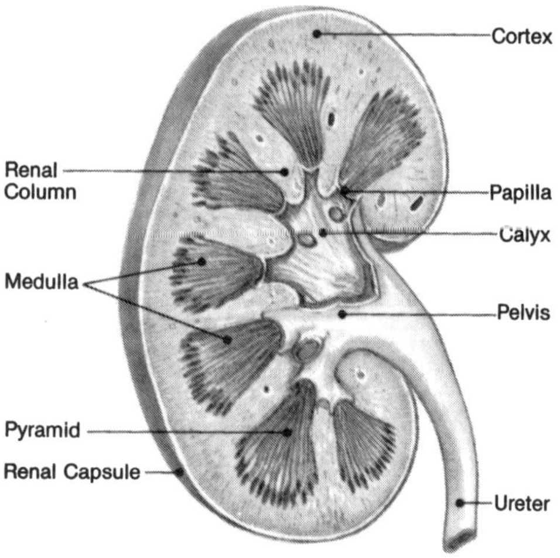

Sectioned Kidney

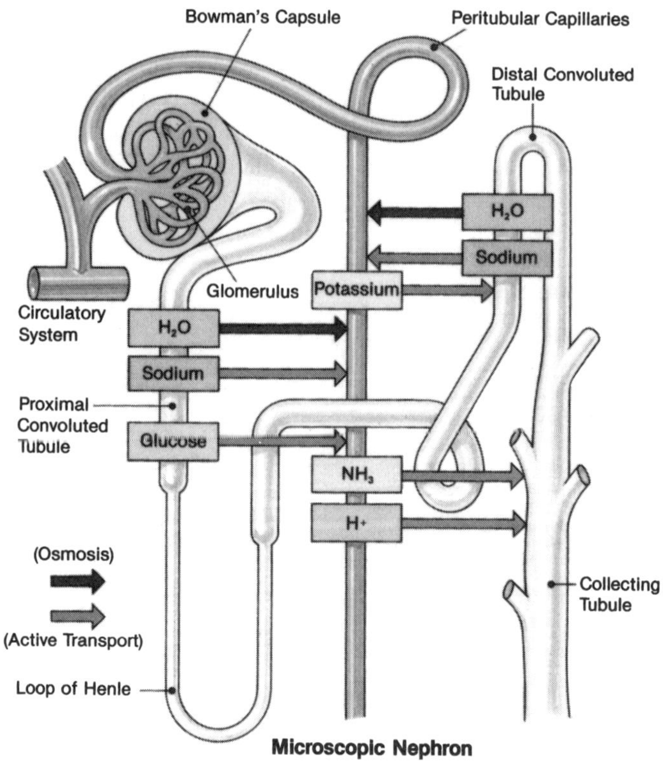

Microscopic Nephron

SOURCE: Harvey D. Grant, et al., Brady Emergency Care, *5th edition, (Englewood Cliffs, NJ: Prentice Hall, 1990) p. 54.*

D

Heat Index

TABLE 1 AIR TEMPERATURE AND RELATIVE HUMIDITY VERSUS APPARENT TEMPERATURE

AIR TEMPERATURE (°F)	Relative Humidity (%) 0	5	10	15	20	25	30	35	40	45	50	55	60	65	70	75	80	85	90	95	100
140	125																				
135	120	128																			
130	117	122	131																		
125	111	116	123	131	141									APPARENT TEMPERATURE							
120	107	111	116	123	130	139	148														
115	103	107	111	115	120	127	135	143	151												
110	99	102	105	108	112	117	123	130	137	143	150										
105	95	97	100	102	105	109	113	118	123	129	135	142	149								
100	91	93	95	97	99	101	104	107	110	115	120	126	132	138	144						
95	87	88	90	91	93	94	96	98	101	104	107	110	114	119	124	130	136				
90	83	84	85	86	87	88	90	91	93	95	96	98	100	102	106	109	113	117	122		
85	78	79	80	81	82	83	84	85	86	87	88	89	90	91	93	95	97	99	102	105	108
80	73	74	75	76	77	77	78	79	79	80	81	81	82	83	85	86	86	87	88	89	91
75	69	69	70	71	72	72	73	73	74	74	75	75	76	76	77	77	78	78	79	79	80
70	64	64	65	65	66	66	67	67	68	68	69	69	70	70	70	70	71	71	71	71	72

Courtesy National Oceanic and Atmospheric Administration

E

Burn Chart

National Burn Information Exchange

I. Feller, M.D., Director, Ann Arbor, Michigan 48104

Form Completed By: ____________________

Name: ____________________

Date: ______________ Age: ______________

Past Medical History: ____________________

Concurrent Injuries: ____________________

Estimation of Size of Burn by Percent

❶ ☐ COLOR IN THE BURN

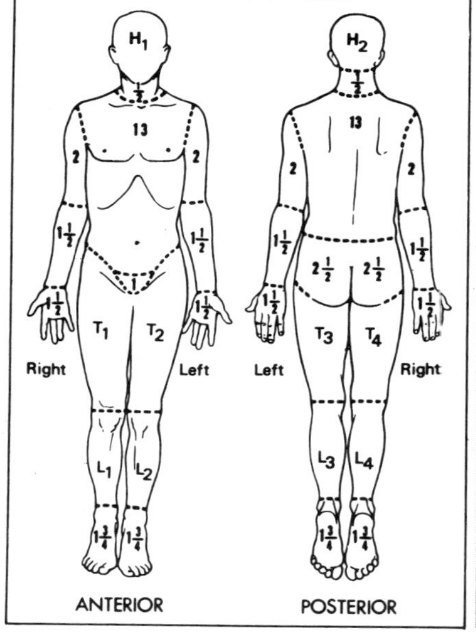

❸ CALCULATE EXTENT BURN

	ANTERIOR	POSTERIOR
Head	H_1 ___	H_2 ___
Neck	___	___
Rt. Arm	___	___
Rt. Forearm	___	___
Rt. Hand	___	___
Lt. Arm	___	___
Lt. Forearm	___	___
Lt. Hand	___	___
Trunk	___	___
Buttock	(R) ___	(L) ___
Perineum	___	___
Rt. Thigh	T_1 ___	T_4 ___
Rt. Leg	L_1 ___	L_4 ___
Rt. Foot	___	___
Lt. Thigh	T_2 ___	T_3 ___
Lt. Leg	L_2 ___	L_3 ___
Lt. Foot	___	___
SUBTOTAL	___	___
% TOTAL AREA BURNED		___ %

❷ CIRCLE AGE FACTOR — PERCENT OF AREAS AFFECTED BY GROWTH

	AGE 0	1	5	10	15	Adult
H(1 or 2) = ½ of the Head	9½	8½	6½	5½	4½	3½
T(1,2,3 or 4) = ½ of a Thigh	2¾	3¼	4	4¼	4½	4¾
L(1,2,3 or 4) = ½ of a Leg	2½	2½	2¾	3	3¼	3½

(see instructions on back)

INSTRUCTIONS FOR COMPLETING THIS FORM

COLOR IN THE BURN

1 Shade or color in the body diagrams to represent as closely as possible how the burn looks to you when viewing the patient from directly anterior and/or directly posterior. Ignore the dashed lines on the diagrams while doing this.

CIRCLE AGE FACTOR

2 Since body proportions change from infancy to adulthood and since these changes mainly affect relative head and lower extremity proportions, this table allows you to choose the most appropriate body proportions for the age of the patient. Ages 0, 1, 5, 10, 15 and adult are given. Choose the age closest to that of the patient and use the H (head), T (thigh) and L (leg) percentage factors in the column below the age selected. To avoid mistakes, circle these numbers.

CALCULATE EXTENT BURN

3 Each body part listed in the calculation table is indicated on the anterior and posterior body diagrams by dashed lines. The percentage of total body surface area for each body part is printed either on the diagram or in the age factor table (step 2). If the shaded or colored area in the body diagram covers an entire body part, the whole percentage figure for that part is entered into the calculation table. If the shaded area covers only a fraction of a body part, then that fraction of the percentage figure is entered. For example, if an anterior chest burn covered about one-third of the trunk, then 1/3 of 13, or 4% would be entered in the space for "trunk (anterior)". When all body parts have been considered, subtotals are made for anterior and posterior burned areas. The grand total then represents an estimate of the percent of total body area burned. This number is most frequently referred to as the "size of burn".

F

Chill Factor

TABLE 10-2 WIND-CHILL FACTOR

Estimated wind speed (in MPH)	Actual Thermometer Reading (°F) 50	40	30	20	10	0	−10	−20	−30	−40	−50	−60
	Equivalent Temperature (°F)											
calm	50	40	30	20	10	0	−10	−20	−30	−40	−50	−60
5	40	37	27	16	6	−5	−15	−26	−36	−47	−57	−68
10	40	28	16	4	−9	−24	−33	−46	−58	−70	−83	−95
15	36	22	9	−5	−18	−32	−45	−58	−72	−85	−99	−112
20	32	18	4	−10	−25	−39	−53	−67	−82	−96	-110	−124
25	30	16	0	−15	−29	−44	−59	−74	−88	−104	−118	−133
30	25	13	−2	−18	−33	−48	−63	−79	−94	−109	−125	−140
35	27	11	−4	−20	−35	−51	−67	−82	−98	−113	−129	−145
40	26	10	−6	−21	−37	−53	−69	−85	−100	−116	−132	−148
(Winds speeds greater than 40 mph have little additional effect.)	Little danger (for properly clothed person). Maximum danger of false sense of security.				Increasing danger (flesh may freeze within 1 minute).			Great danger (flesh may freeze within 30 seconds).				

Source: Grant and Murray, Emergency Care *(Bowie, Md.: Robert J. Brady Co., 1978).*

G

Dive Chart

*The following is a brief description of the standard use of the NAVY Dive Charts. These charts are time limits that are based on young physically fit males. For this reason, calculation should round up rather than using exact figures.

Table 1 is used when there is a non-decompression dive or when a dive exceeds the Bottom Time Interval. The far left-hand columns are used for the no-decompression dive. Once the time limit in the second left-hand column is exceeded, a group designation is gained (through the use of Table 3).

Table 2 is used for repetitive dives. This chart will establish group designation for repetitive dives and surface time intervals.

Table 3 describes decompression time factors and the associated decompression depth along with end group designation.

TABLE 1 SPORT DIVER OPEN WATER U.S. NAVY DIVE TABLES

No-decompression limits and repetitive group designation table for no-decompression air dives

Depth (feet)	No-decom-pression limits (min)	Group Designation A	B	C	D	E	F	G	H	I	J	K	L	M	N	O
10		60	120	210	300											
15		35	70	110	160	225	350									
20		25	50	75	100	135	180	240	325							
25	(245)	20	35	55	75	100	125	160	195	245	315					
30	(205)	15	30	45	60	75	95	120	145	170	205	250	310			
35	(160) 310	5	15	25	40	50	60	80	100	120	140	160	190	220	270	310
40	(130) 200	5	15	25	30	40	50	70	80	100	110	130	150	170	200	
50	(70) 100		10	15	25	30	40	50	60	70	80	90	100			
60	(50) 60		10	15	20	25	30	40	50	55	60					
70	(40) 50		5	10	15	20	30	35	40	45	50					
80	(30) 40		5	10	15	20	25	30	35	40						
90	(25) 30		5	10	12	15	20	25	30							
100	(20) 25		5	7	10	15	20	22	25							
110	(15) 20			5	10	13	15	20								
120	(10) 15			5	10	12	15									
130	(5) 10			5	8	10										
140	10			5	7	10										

No Decompression — Residual Nitrogen levels

TABLE 2 RESIDUAL NITROGEN TIMETABLE FOR REPETITIVE AIR DIVES

Repetitive group at the beginning of the surface interval	Z	O	N	M	L	K	J	I	H	G	F	E	D	C	B	A
A																0:10 12:00*
B															0:10 2:10	2:11 12:00*
C														0:10 1:39	1:40 2:49	2:50 12:00*
D													0:10 1:09	1:10 2:38	2:39 5:48	5:49 12:00*
E												0:10 0:54	0:55 1:57	1:58 3:22	3:23 6:32	6:33 12:00*
F											0:10 0:45	0:46 1:29	1:30 2:28	2:29 3:57	3:58 7:05	7:06 12:00*
G										0:10 0:40	0:41 1:15	1:16 1:59	2:00 2:58	2:59 4:25	4:26 7:35	7:36 12:00*
H									0:10 0:36	0:37 1:06	1:07 1:41	1:42 2:23	2:24 3:20	3:21 4:49	4:50 7:59	8:00 12:00*
I								0:10 0:33	0:34 0:59	1:00 1:29	1:30 2:02	2:03 2:44	2:45 3:43	3:44 5:12	5:13 8:21	8:22 12:00*
J							0:10 0:31	0:32 0:54	0:55 1:19	1:20 1:47	1:48 2:20	2:21 3:04	3:05 4:02	4:03 5:40	5:41 8:40	8:41 12:00*
K						0:10 0:28	0:29 0:49	0:50 1:11	1:12 1:35	1:36 2:03	2:04 2:38	2:39 3:21	3:22 4:19	4:20 5:48	5:49 8:58	8:59 12:00*
L					0:10 0:26	0:27 0:45	0:46 1:04	1:05 1:25	1:26 1:49	1:50 2:19	2:20 2:53	2:54 3:36	3:37 4:35	4:36 6:02	6:03 9:12	9:13 12:00*
M				0:10 0:25	0:26 0:42	0:43 0:59	1:00 1:18	1:19 1:39	1:40 2:05	2:06 2:34	2:35 3:08	3:09 3:52	3:53 4:49	4:50 6:18	6:19 9:28	9:29 12:00*
N			0:10 0:24	0:25 0:39	0:40 0:54	0:55 1:11	1:12 1:30	1:31 1:53	1:54 2:18	2:19 2:47	2:48 3:22	3:23 4:04	4:05 5:03	5:04 6:32	6:33 9:43	9:44 12:00*
O		0:10 0:23	0.24 0:36	0:37 0:51	0:52 1:07	1:08 1:24	1:25 1:43	1:44 2:04	2:05 2:29	2:30 2:59	3:00 3:33	3:34 4:17	4:18 5:16	5:17 6.44	6:45 9:54	9:55 12:00*
Z	0:10 0:22	0:23 0:34	0:35 0:48	0:49 1:02	1:03 1:18	1:19 1:36	1:37 1:55	1:56 2:17	2:18 2:42	2:43 3:10	3:11 3:45	3:46 4:29	4:30 5:27	5:28 6:56	6:57 10:05	10:06 12:00*

NEW→ GROUP DESIGNATION / REPETITIVE DIVE DEPTH	Z	O	N	M	L	K	J	I	H	G	F	E	D	C	B	A
40	257	241	213	187	161	138	116	101	87	73	61	49	37	25	17	7
50	169	160	142	124	111	99	87	76	66	56	47	38	29	21	13	6
60	122	117	107	97	88	79	70	61	52	44	36	30	24	17	11	5
70	100	96	87	80	72	64	57	50	43	37	31	26	20	15	9	4
80	84	80	73	68	61	54	48	43	38	32	28	23	18	13	8	4
90	73	70	64	58	53	47	43	38	33	29	24	20	16	11	7	3
100	64	62	57	52	48	43	38	34	30	26	22	18	14	10	7	3
110	57	55	51	47	42	38	34	31	27	24	20	16	13	10	6	3
120	52	50	46	43	39	35	32	28	25	21	18	15	12	9	6	3
130	46	44	40	38	35	31	28	25	22	19	16	13	11	8	6	3
140	42	40	38	35	32	29	26	23	20	18	15	12	10	7	5	2

Residual nitrogen times (minutes)

TABLE 3 NAVY STANDARD AIR DECOMPRESSION TABLE

Depth (feet)	Bottom time (min)	Time first stop (min:sec)	Decompression stops (feet)		Total ascent (min:sec)	Repetitive group
			20	10		
40	200			0	0:40	*
	210	0:30		2	2:40	N
	230	0:30		7	7:40	N
	250	0:30		11	11:40	O
50	100			0	0:50	*
	110	0:40		3	3:50	L
	120	0:40		5	5:50	M
	140	0:40		10	10:50	M
	160	0:40		21	21:50	N
60	60			0	1:00	*
	70	0:50		2	3:00	K
	80	0:50		7	8:00	L
	100	0:50		14	15:00	M
	120	0:50		26	27:00	N
70	50			0	1:10	*
	60	1:00		8	9:10	K
	70	1:00		14	15:10	L
	80	1:00		18	19:10	M
	90	1:00		23	24:10	N
80	40			0	1:20	*
	50	1:10		10	11:20	K
	60	1:10		17	18:20	L
	70	1:10		23	24:20	M
90	30			0	1:30	*
	40	1:20		7	8:30	J
	50	1:20		18	19:30	L
	60	1:20		25	26:30	M
100	25			0	1:40	*
	30	1:30		3	4:40	I
	40	1:30		15	16:40	K
	50	1:20	2	24	27:40	L
110	20			0	1:50	*
	25	1:40		3	4:50	H
	30	1:40		7	8:50	J
	40	1:30	2	21	24:50	L
120	15			0	2:00	*
	20	1:50		2	4:00	H
	25	1:50		6	8:00	I
	30	1:50		14	16:00	J
130	10			0	2:10	*
	15	2:00		1	3:10	F
	20	2:00		4	6:10	H
	25	2:00		10	12:10	J
140	10			0	2:20	*
	15	2:10		2	4:20	G
	20	2:10		6	8:20	I
	25	2:00	2	14	18:20	J

Source: U.S. Navy dive charts.

H

Oxygen Charts: Standards of Volume

All charts are based on 500 lbs of residual pressure. The intersection of pressure in the tank and liters per minute gives a resultant of minutes left in the oxygen cylinder.

D-SIZE CYLINDER

Pressure in tank	2	4	6	8	10	11	12	13	14	15
	Liters per minute									
2000	120	60	40	30	24	22	20	18	17	16
1975	118	59	39	30	24	21	20	18	17	16
1950	116	58	39	29	23	21	19	18	17	15
1925	114	57	38	29	23	21	19	18	16	15
1900	112	56	37	28	22	20	19	17	16	15
1875	110	55	37	28	22	20	18	17	16	15
1850	108	54	36	27	22	20	18	17	15	14
1825	106	53	35	27	21	19	18	16	15	14
1800	104	52	35	26	21	19	17	16	15	14
1775	102	51	34	26	20	19	17	16	15	14
1750	100	50	33	25	20	18	17	15	14	13
1725	98	49	33	25	20	18	16	15	14	13
1700	96	48	32	24	19	17	16	15	14	13
1675	94	47	31	24	19	17	16	14	13	13
1650	92	46	31	23	18	17	15	14	13	12
1625	90	45	30	23	18	16	15	14	13	12
1600	88	44	29	22	18	16	15	14	13	12
1575	86	43	29	22	17	16	14	13	12	11
1550	84	42	28	21	17	15	14	13	12	11
1525	82	41	27	21	16	15	14	13	12	11
1500	80	40	27	20	16	15	13	12	11	11
1475	78	39	26	20	16	14	13	12	11	10
1450	76	38	25	19	15	14	13	12	11	10
1425	74	37	25	19	15	13	12	11	11	10
1400	72	36	24	18	14	13	12	11	10	10
1375	70	35	23	18	14	13	12	11	10	9
1350	68	34	23	17	14	12	11	10	10	9
1325	66	33	22	17	13	12	11	10	9	9
1300	64	32	21	16	13	12	11	10	9	9
1275	62	31	21	16	12	11	10	10	9	8
1250	60	30	20	15	12	11	10	9	9	8
1225	58	29	19	15	12	11	10	9	8	8
1200	56	28	19	14	11	10	9	9	8	7
1175	54	27	18	14	11	10	9	8	8	7
1150	52	26	17	13	10	9	9	8	7	7
1125	50	25	17	13	10	9	8	8	7	7
1100	48	24	16	12	10	9	8	7	7	6
1075	46	23	15	12	9	8	8	7	7	6
1050	44	22	15	11	9	8	7	7	6	6
1025	42	21	14	11	8	8	7	6	6	6
1000	40	20	13	10	8	7	7	6	6	5
975	38	19	13	10	8	7	6	6	5	5
950	36	18	12	9	7	7	6	6	5	5

925	34	17	11	9	7	6	6	5	5	5
900	32	16	11	8	6	6	5	5	5	4
875	30	15	10	8	6	5	5	5	4	4
850	28	14	9	7	6	5	5	4	4	4
825	26	13	9	7	5	5	4	4	4	3
800	24	12	8	6	5	4	4	4	3	3
775	22	11	7	6	4	4	4	3	3	3
750	20	10	7	5	4	4	3	3	3	3
725	18	9	6	5	4	3	3	3	3	2
700	16	8	5	4	3	3	3	2	2	2
675	14	7	5	4	3	3	2	2	2	2
650	12	6	4	3	2	2	2	2	2	2
625	10	5	3	3	2	2	2	2	1	1
600	8	4	3	2	2	1	1	1	1	1
575	6	3	2	2	1	1	1	1	1	1
550	4	2	1	1	1	1	1	1	1	1
525	2	1	1	1	0	0	C	0	0	0

E-SIZE CYLINDER

Pressure in tank	2	4	6	8	10	11	12	13	14	15
	Liters per minute									
2000	210	105	70	53	42	38	35	32	30	28
1975	207	103	69	52	41	38	34	32	30	28
1950	203	102	68	51	41	37	34	31	29	27
1925	200	100	67	50	40	36	33	31	29	27
1900	196	98	65	49	39	36	33	30	28	26
1875	193	96	64	48	39	35	32	30	28	26
1850	189	95	63	47	38	34	32	29	27	25
1825	186	93	62	46	37	34	31	29	27	25
1800	182	91	61	46	36	33	30	28	26	24
1775	179	89	60	45	36	32	30	27	26	24
1750	175	88	58	44	35	32	29	27	25	23
1725	172	86	57	43	34	31	29	26	25	23
1700	168	84	56	42	34	31	28	26	24	22
1675	165	82	55	41	33	30	27	25	24	22
1650	161	81	54	40	32	29	27	25	23	21
1625	158	79	53	39	32	29	26	24	23	21
1600	154	77	51	39	31	28	26	24	22	21
1575	151	75	50	38	30	27	25	23	22	20
1550	147	74	49	37	29	27	25	23	21	20
1525	144	72	48	36	29	26	24	22	21	19
1500	140	70	47	35	28	25	23	22	20	19
1475	137	68	46	34	27	25	23	21	20	18
1450	133	67	44	33	27	24	22	20	19	18
1425	130	65	43	32	26	24	22	20	19	17
1400	126	63	42	32	25	23	21	19	18	17
1375	123	61	41	31	25	22	20	19	18	16
1350	119	60	40	30	24	22	20	18	17	16
1325	116	58	39	29	23	21	19	18	17	15
1300	112	56	37	28	22	20	19	17	16	15
1275	109	54	36	27	22	20	18	17	16	14
1250	105	53	35	26	21	19	18	16	15	14
1225	102	51	34	25	20	18	17	16	15	14
1200	98	49	33	25	20	18	16	15	14	13
1175	95	47	32	24	19	17	16	15	14	13
1150	91	46	30	23	18	17	15	14	13	12
1125	88	44	29	22	18	16	15	13	13	12
1100	84	42	28	21	17	15	14	13	12	11
1075	81	40	27	20	16	15	13	12	12	11
1050	77	39	26	19	15	14	13	12	11	10
1025	74	37	25	18	15	13	12	11	11	10
1000	70	35	23	18	14	13	12	11	10	9
975	67	33	22	17	13	12	11	10	10	9

950	63	32	21	16	13	11	11	10	9	8
925	60	30	20	15	12	11	10	9	9	8
900	56	28	19	14	11	10	9	9	8	7
875	53	26	18	13	11	10	9	8	8	7
850	49	25	16	12	10	9	8	8	7	7
825	46	23	15	11	9	8	8	7	7	6
800	42	21	14	11	8	8	7	6	6	6
775	39	19	13	10	8	7	6	6	6	5
750	35	18	12	9	7	6	6	5	5	5
725	32	16	11	8	6	6	5	5	5	4
700	28	14	9	7	6	5	5	4	4	4
675	25	12	8	6	5	4	4	4	4	3
650	21	11	7	5	4	4	4	3	3	3
625	18	9	6	4	4	3	3	3	3	2
600	14	7	5	4	3	3	2	2	2	2
575	11	5	4	3	2	2	2	2	2	1
550	7	4	2	2	1	1	1	1	1	1
525	4	2	1	1	1	1	1	1	1	0

M-SIZE CYLINDER

Pressure in tank	2	4	6	8	10	11	12	13	14	15
					Liters per minute					
2000	1170	585	390	293	234	213	195	180	167	156
1975	1151	575	384	288	230	209	192	177	164	153
1950	1131	565	377	283	226	206	189	174	162	151
1925	1112	556	371	278	222	202	185	171	159	148
1900	1092	546	364	273	218	199	182	168	156	146
1875	1073	536	358	268	215	195	179	165	153	143
1850	1053	526	351	263	211	191	176	162	150	140
1825	1034	517	345	258	207	188	172	159	148	138
1800	1014	507	338	254	203	184	169	156	145	135
1775	994	497	332	249	199	181	166	153	142	133
1750	975	487	325	244	195	177	163	150	139	130
1725	955	478	319	239	191	174	159	147	137	127
1700	936	468	312	234	187	170	156	144	134	125
1675	916	458	306	229	183	167	153	141	131	122
1650	897	448	299	224	179	163	150	138	128	120
1625	877	439	293	219	176	160	146	135	125	117
1600	858	429	286	215	172	156	143	132	123	114
1575	838	419	280	210	168	152	140	129	120	112
1550	819	410	273	205	164	149	137	126	117	109
1525	799	400	267	200	160	145	133	123	114	107
1500	780	390	260	195	156	142	130	120	111	104
1475	760	380	254	190	152	138	127	117	109	101
1450	741	371	247	185	148	135	124	114	106	99
1425	721	361	241	180	144	131	120	111	103	96
1400	702	351	234	176	140	128	117	108	100	94
1375	682	341	228	171	137	124	114	105	97	91
1350	663	332	221	166	133	121	111	102	95	88
1325	643	322	215	161	129	117	107	99	92	86
1300	624	312	208	156	125	113	104	96	89	83
1275	604	302	202	151	121	110	101	93	86	81
1250	585	293	195	146	117	106	97	90	84	78
1225	565	283	189	141	113	103	94	87	81	75
1200	546	273	182	137	109	99	91	84	78	73
1175	526	263	176	132	105	96	88	81	75	70
1150	507	254	169	127	101	92	84	78	72	68
1125	487	244	163	122	97	89	81	75	70	65
1100	468	234	156	117	94	85	78	72	67	62
1075	448	224	150	112	90	82	75	69	64	60
1050	429	215	143	107	86	78	71	66	61	57
1025	409	205	137	102	82	74	68	63	59	55
1000	390	195	130	97	78	71	65	60	56	52
975	370	185	124	93	74	67	62	57	53	49
950	351	176	117	88	70	64	58	54	50	47

925	331	166	111	83	66	60	55	51	47	44
900	312	156	104	78	62	57	52	48	45	42
875	292	146	97	73	58	53	49	45	42	39
850	273	137	91	68	55	50	46	42	39	36
825	254	127	85	63	51	46	42	39	36	34
800	234	117	78	59	47	43	39	36	33	31
775	215	107	72	54	43	39	36	33	31	29
750	195	98	65	49	39	35	33	30	28	26
725	176	88	59	44	35	32	29	27	25	23
700	156	78	52	39	31	28	26	24	22	21
675	137	68	46	34	27	25	23	21	20	18
650	117	59	39	29	23	21	20	18	17	16
625	97	49	33	24	20	18	16	15	14	13
600	78	39	26	20	16	14	13	12	11	10
575	59	29	20	15	12	11	10	9	8	8
550	39	20	13	10	8	7	6	6	6	5
525	20	10	6	5	4	4	3	3	3	3

I

Example of SOP for Report Writing

The following is the standard operating procedure (SOP) for writing a medical report. It is an example of all the elements that have been outlined in this book. An example of the report to which the SOP refers is included.

STANDARD OPERATING EMS PROCEDURES

Related EMS Functions

220.0 ***EMS REPORTS***

220.1 ***PURPOSE***
This procedure is designed to establish an information base for the completion of the Trauma Report, and Trauma Registry Scorecard. It is intended to give additional information such that a concise, complete, and well-documented report can be generated.

220.2 ***POLICY***
All field operations personnel shall know how to fully document an EMS incident. The responsibility for completion of the report resides with the engineer and or lieutenant in charge; however, the task may be delegated to a lower rank (BSO-87-915-12; 4.0). All Trauma Reports and Trauma Registry forms shall be filled out in black ink.

220.3 ***DESCRIPTION***
When completing the Trauma Report (Orange County 40-1), three documents shall be used as reference:
.1 Completion of UFIRS Reports CM-916-88-3.

.2 First Aid/EMS Trauma Reports BSO-87-915-12.

.3 Orange County EMS System Standing Orders.

221.0 Upon completion, the Trauma Reports shall be mailed through the interdepartmental mail system to the Records/Reports Section.

.1 All incidents shall have a report generated before a duty tour is completed.

.2 All Trauma Reports shall utilize the CHARTE format for documentation (see EMS SOP 223.2).

.2.1 C—Chief Complaint

.2.2 H—History

.2.3 A—Assessment: head-to-toe survey

.2.4 R—Treatment: time line may be utilized

.2.5 T—Transport: document all activity while enroute to the hospital if OFD personnel accompany the patient to the medical facility

.2.6 E—Exceptions

222.0 All Trauma Reports shall be received at the Records/Reports Section within 72 hours after completion of the shift. The report shall be reviewed for completeness, legibility, and proper treatment of the situation. If a report is found to have a discrepancy, it shall be sent back to the writer for correction. After completion, the EMS office shall again review the report.

.1 When a discrepancy is found, the sender is notified.

.1.2 The sender shall correct the problem by correction on an additional Trauma Report. Not all information need be on the new report.

.1.2.1 identifying information and the correction.

.1.2.2 Boxes 1, 7, 8, 11, 12, 13, 35, 36, signature, and date.

.1.3 This new addition is sent to the EMS office.

223.0 Completion of Incident Reports: See BSO-87-915-12; 3.0

.1 Biographical information: data required

.1.1 Box 1: Patient's name—Print patient's full name.

.1.2 Box 2: Sex—Enter the gender of the patient using the following abbreviations: M = male and F = female.

.1.3 Box 3: Date of birth or age—Enter the patient's date of birth if birthdate is available, or age if birthdate is unavailable.

.1.4 Box 4: Race—Enter B = black, C = Caucasian, H = Hispanic, O = other.

.1.5 Box 5: Weight—Enter weight in kilograms (dividing patient's weight in pounds by 2 gives an approximate weight in kilograms).

.1.6 Box 6: Res—If patient is a resident of Orange County, enter "Y" for yes and "N" for no.

.1.6.1 Private physician—Enter patient's physician's name if known. If patient has a certain medical problem, enter the name of the physician who is taking care of that condition.

.1.7 Box 7: Patient's address—Enter patient's street address, including zip code. If the street address is unknown, enter "unknown."

.1.8 Box 8: Run number—Enter Orlando Fire Department's computer-generated alarm number assigned to the incident.

.1.9 Box 9: Patient number—Enter the patient number relative to the number of patients. Example: If the incident has five patients and you are treating patient 3, enter 3/5. Number in order of transport.

.1.10 Box 10: Agy—Letter assigned by Orange County to designate the agency generating the report. Enter "K" for Orlando Fire Department.

.1.11 Box 11: Stn—Enter the station number of the unit generating the report, using left-hand justification. Example: Rescue 2 would enter "02."

.1.11.1 Unit—Number designation of the unit generating the report.

.1.11.2 Rescue Companies = 100 series.

.1.11.3 Engine Companies = 200 series.

.1.11.4 Tower Companies = 300 series.

.1.11.5 Any company that is manned in addition to the normal city fire force, such as reserve equipment placed into primary response = 400 series.

.1.11.6 Second house rescue, engine, or tower shall enumerate the appropriate series with the ten's placeholder designating the number. Example: Engine 101 = 221; 200 being the Engine Company, 21 showing that it is the second engine within Station 1.

.1.11.7 Dest. Det.: Destination Determined—Enter the applicable letter as indicated by the listing on the back of the Trauma Report.

.1.12 Box 12: Incident Location—Enter the street address where the patient is being treated. This may not be the same as the location where the incident was dispatched. Building names or landmarks are not acceptable. Intersections or divided highways, with direction of travel and nearest access ramp as location, are acceptable.

.1.13 Box 13: Run Date—Date on which the incident occurred. Enter mm/dd/yy.

.1.14 Box 14: S.T.R.—Section, Township, and Range as indicated on the STR map.

.1.15 Box 15: Dup.—Enter "Y" if another EMS agency responded to the incident and will also complete an Orange County Trauma Report. Enter "N" if no other EMS agency responds.

.1.15.1 Police—Enter abbreviation of law enforcement agency that responds.
Orange County Sheriff's Office = OCSO
Orlando Police Department = OPD
Florida Highway Patrol = FHP

.1.16 Box 16: Call Rec'd—Enter time call received as indicated on the computer alarm history.

.1.17 Box 17: Unit Enrt.—Enter time unit enroute to the incident as indicated on the computer alarm history.

.1.18 Box 18: Arr'vd LOC—Enter time unit arrives on the scene as indicated by the computer alarm history.

.1.19 Box 19: Arr'vd Pt—Enter the estimated time the crew actually gets to the patient. This data must be noted on the scene; it is not captured by dispatch.

.1.20 Box 20: Pt. Dep'd—Enter the estimated time the patient departs the scene. Enter data here only when the patient departs by an EMS transporting agency. This information must be noted by on-scene personnel.

.1.21 Box 21: Arr'vd Dest.—Enter the estimated time the patient arrives at the hospital when Orlando Fire Department accompanied the patient to the hospital.

.1.22 Box 22: Unit Avail.—Enter the time the unit is available for another alarm. Data is available on the computer alarm history.

.1.23 Box 23: Mileage—Entry here is required only if the unit arrives on the scene. Enter only mileage to the scene unless Orlando Fire Department transports the patient to the hospital.

.1.24 Box 24: Type of call—Enter "A" if the unit responds to the scene emergency. Enter "B" if the unit responds to the scene nonemergency. Enter "C" if a public service; a MODULE 2 will also have to be generated.

.1.25 Box 25: Disp. of Call—Enter the appropriate letter that corresponds with the disposition of the patient (see the listing on the reverse side of the Trauma Report).

.1.25.1 Standby—Indicates that a bona fide incident exists but services were not utilized (standby for hostage situation).

.1.25.2 Dry Run—Indicates that an incident exists but services are not rendered (auto accident where occupants deny injury, patient has left scene).

.1.25.3 If patients on scene deny injury, consider medical release form signed and documented.

.1.26 Box 26: Pt. Taken to—Enter the letter that corresponds with the facility to which the patient was taken (see the listing on the reverse side of the Trauma Report).

.1.27 Box 27: Extrication—Enter the estimated time taken to extricate the patient in hours and minutes. Extrication from entanglement, not necessarily auto, could be from any container. This is the amount of time in minutes.

.1.28 Box 28: Seatbelts—Enter "Y" if the patient is observed wearing seatbelt. *The patient must be observed.* Enter "N" if the patient is not observed wearing a seatbelt. If the patient, law enforcement officer, or other person *states* that seatbelts were in place but were removed prior to OFD observing, enter "N" or S/R and make a notation in the comments section about such statements.

.1.29 Box 29: Child Restraints—Enter "Y" if yes and "N" if no. Follow the guidelines outlined for 28.

.1.30 Box 30: Helmet—Enter "Y" if yes and "N" if no. Use the guidelines outlined in box 28.

.1.31 Box 31: Anatomy of Injury—Enter the letter corresponding to the anatomy (mechanism) of injury the patient presents. Use the listing provided on the back of the Trauma Report. If none of the listed anatomies of injury apply, strike through the box.

.1.32 Box 32: Glascow Coma Score—Compute trauma score using criteria on the back of the Trauma Report, and enter the total. Scores range from 3 to 15. Any patient presenting with a score of less than 13 is to be transported to a Level 1 Trauma Center.

.1.33 Box 33: Nature of Run—Enter the letter corresponding to the nature of the incident found on arrival. *On all codes:* Enter "XX"for a patient save (any patient delivered to the E.R. who has a viable rhythm), or "Z" if the patient is pronounced D.O.A. at the hospital or scene.

.1.34 Box 34: Protocol Used—Enter the letter that corresponds to the protocol required by the patient's presenting signs and symptoms. Multiple protocols may be entered (up to 7). All ALS incidents must utilize a specific protocol. Standing orders may not be entered as the sole protocol used. If a physician's orders ("B") are entered, a notation in the comments section must reflect the orders given. If a prophylactic IV is initiated, enter S/R in this box and make a notation regarding the circumstances in the comments section. A list of signs and symptoms shall be noted along with how the patient presented.

.1.34.1 Allergies—Enter all known allergies the patient may have (medical, food, insect, etc.)

.1.34.2. Report Received—Have the person accepting a copy of the report at the hospital enter his or her signature here. If the signature is not available, enter the name of the person receiving the report copy.

.1.34.3 Physician's Sign—Have the attending physician or his or her designee sign here. If the physician or designee cannot sign, enter his or her name here. All records utilizing physician's orders shall have a doctor's signature.

.1.35 Box 35: Attendant A—Enter the name and PM number of the OFD crew member writing the report.

.1.36 Box 36: Attendant B—Enter the name and PM number of the OFD crew member who assisted attendant A.

.1.37 Box 37: Other—Enter the names, unit number, and/or agency name that assisted with patient care.

.1.38 Box 38: Other—Enter the names, unit number, and/or agency name that assisted with patient care. To differentiate between Other in box 37 and box 38, an Other 1 and Other 2 (or Other A or Other B) may be used.

.1.39 Box 39: ALS—Enter "Y" if ALS measures were initiated and "N" if they were not. A quick look with the EKG paddles is *not* considered an ALS measure but rather, a diagnostic tool.

.1.40 Box 40: Arrythmia—Enter the corresponding number of the patient's initial presenting rhythm. A listing is provided on the back of the Trauma Report. All rhythms presented by the patient shall be enumerated in the time line as well as documented with a 6-second strip for each rhythm presented. Do not refer to another agency's report. If the strip is lost or destroyed, simply note in the comments section under exceptions (E). Attach the EKG strip to the back of the first Trauma Report and copy. Each strip shall contain the following written information: the patient's name, alarm number, the date, the time, and the attendents' names.

.1.40.1 Two copies of each 6-second strip shall be attached to the Trauma Report: one 6-second strip to the original report, and one attached to the second page. Both are attached to the *back* of each page.

.2 Documentation of Treatment: Comments Section—Enter a brief description of the scene upon arrival. Enter the patient assessment findings and treatment using the CHARTE method.

.2.1 *C:* CHIEF COMPLAINT—Information that the patient tells you. Scene description can be included in this section.

.2.2 *H:* HISTORY OF THE CHIEF COMPLAINT—Record all information regarding the onset, duration, and cause of aggravating factors relative to the chief complaint. Record any medical history the patient may have.

.2.3 *A:* ASSESSMENT—Record all positive and negative findings from the primary and secondary assessments. *Should include a head-to-toe assessment.*

.2.4 *R:* TREATMENT—Record all treatment provided to the patient while in your care.

.2.5 *T:* TRANSPORTATION—Record to where the patient was transported and by whom.

.2.6 *E:* EXCEPTIONS—Record any deviations from protocol or SOP. All S/R entries should also receive explanation here.

.2.7 Trauma Registry Number—Shall be placed in the lower right-hand corner of the comments section.

.3 Time Line of Patient Care—This section is to be completed in the sequence of treatment.

.3.1 Time—Enter the estimated time when specific treatment rendered.

.3.2 LOC—Enter the level of consciousness the patient demonstrated throughout his or her care.

.3.3 B/P, P, R—Enter the blood pressure, pulse, and respirations of the patient. Vitals are for that specific time only; all vitals are to be reassessed every 5 minutes on ALS patients.

.3.4 CC/EKG—Enter the condition or arrhythmia being treated. When EKG changes, it shall be noted in this box with attached 6-second strip.

.3.5 TREATMENT—Enter the treatment rendered (see documentation suggestions).

.3.6 RESPONSE—Enter the patient's response to the treatment rendered (see documentation suggestions).

.3.7 AID/ATT—Enter the letter that corresponds to the treatment provided as listed on the back of the trauma report. Also enter the attendant rendering the aid.

.3.8 Signature and Date—The person whose name appears as attendant "A" must sign and date the report here.

.4 Miscellaneous Information:

.4.1 Reports are to be completed before the end of the tour of duty on which the incident occurred.

.4.2 Reports are to be completed in black ink.
.5 Patient refusal forms:
.5.1 Fill out on all patients who refuse treatment and/or transportation.
.5.2 Forms must contain the following information:
.5.2.1 Patient's name.
.5.2.2 Patient's home address.
.5.2.3 Incident location.
.5.2.4 Agency designation.
.5.2.5 Alarm number and date.
.5.2.6 Reason for refusal, notification/ramifications of not seeking medical attention, vitals if appropriate, and refusal in front of witnesses.
.5.2.7 Documentation of refusal:
.5.2.7.1 Patient must be made aware of the consequences of the incident.
.5.2.7.2 Patient understood the consequences stated.
.5.2.7.3 Patient made a verbal response of the above in front of witnesses.
.5.3 Check appropriate box describing patient's refusal of services.
.5.4 If multiple patients at a single incident location: For all the patients who refuse service, complete a single Trauma Report with the following data:
.5.4.1 Complete boxes 8–40 (box 9 should be completed with 1/1 entered). Some entries may not always be applicable; if not, strike through the box.
.5.4.2 List in the comments section the names of each patient refusing services and make a notation that all patients have refused services. Make a note if a specific service was refused.
.5.4.3 Complete a patient refusal form for *each* patient, entering all patient data requested on the refusal form. Have each patient sign and date the appropriate form.
.5.5 Attach the refusal form(s) to the back of the first page of the Trauma Report.

224.0 In 1987 the state legislature enacted the Trauma Care Act. The law was established in order to view how trauma is handled throughout the state. The sole purpose of the registry is to evaluate the trauma care currently being delivered in the state of Florida. It will assess the care of EMS providers, trauma centers, pediatric trauma referral centers, and hospitals.

225.0 To answer the questions posed, the state devised a form that will track a trauma patient from the scene to the hospital.
.1 100% compliance is essential. It is an absolute must that parts 1 and 2 of state form 1729 shall be completed prior to transport.
.1.1 The law states that a Trauma Form (HRS-Form *1728*) shall be completed on all trauma victims (for a definition of trauma, see 215.3 and 215.3.1).
.1.2 This form shall accompany the patient to the hospital.
.2 Parts 1 and 2 shall be completed by the EMS first-response provider.

.2.1 This form must be completed prior to transportation.
.2.2 Pages 1, 2, and 3 shall be handed to the transporting agency.
.2.3 Page 4 is attached to the Trauma Report.
.3 Anyone who has sustained a blunt or penetrating injury and is transported to ORMC shall have a Trauma Scorecard filled out (see Appendix B).
.3.1 Exception: Trauma patients pronounced dead on scene. This shall follow Orange County SOP.

226.0 The form is in four pages on NCR paper. The bottom copy shall remain with the EMS provider (Rescue or Engine/Tower). The top three copies shall follow the patient to the hospital.
.1 Staple the bottom page of the state registry to the Trauma Report and forward to the Records/Report Section.

227.0 The responsibility for the completion of the Trauma Scorecard shall be with the PM II on Rescue and the Lieutenant on Engine and/or Tower.
.1 When the Orlando Fire Department transports, Rescue is responsible for completion of the Orange County Trauma Report and Trauma Scorecard.

228.0 General Instructions for the Trauma Scorecard
.1 This form is to be typed or printed in black ink.
.1.1 Times must be entered in military time format.
.1.2 Dates must be entered in mm/dd/yy format.
.2 Complete the form for:
.2.1 Trauma victims.
.2.2 Head injury victims.
.2.3 Spinal cord victims.
.2.4 Spinal cord disease victims and cases of blindness or amputation that are required to be reported to Central Registry.
.3 Patient information:
.3.1 Patient's Name—Last name, first name; if name is unknown enter "unknown."
.3.2 Age—Actual or estimated age of the patient; if less than 1 year, enter zero (0).
.3.3 Race—Check applicable box.
.3.4 Sex—Check "M" for male, "F" for female.
.3.5 Date of Injury—Enter the date of the injury with left-hand justification.
.3.6 Time of Injury—Enter the appropriate time of injury.
.4 Trauma Scorecard (see Appendix B).
.4.1 Run Report—Enter the alarm number.
.4.2 Time Arrived at Scene—The time the first EMS unit arrived on the scene.
.4.3 Time Alert Called—Enter the time when EMS notified the trauma center of the incoming trauma patient.
.4.3.1 Notification shall be through MEDCOM.
.4.4 Fractures—Indicate whether the trauma victim has suspected bone fracture.
.4.5 Blood Pressure—The initial unassisted blood pressure obtained by the first paramedic or EMT on the scene.

.4.6 Resp. Rate—Respiratory rate; this is the initial assessment by the first paramedic or EMT on the scene.
.4.7 Glasgow Coma Scale Score—Check the appropriate box in each category. Total the numbers checked in each section and write total score in the space marked "total" (see Appendix B).
.4.8 Anatomy of Injury—Check all that apply.
.4.8.1 Steering Wheel Deformed—Indicate if the steering wheel had been deformed.
.4.8.2 Intubated—Indicate if the trauma victim has been intubated and indicate the reason for intubation.
.4.8.2.1 Airway obstructed.
.4.8.2.2 Hyperventilate.
.4.8.2.3 Transport.
.4.8.2.4 Other.
.4.8.3 Protective Devices—Check all appropriate boxes to indicate use of protective devices.
.4.8.4 Cause of Injury—Check applicable cause.
.4.8.5 Fluids—Check the box next to the fluid given and indicate the amount given. D5W and .45 NaCl shall be checked for D5W.
.4.8.6 Medication—List all medications given to the trauma victim and the amount of the dosage.
.4.8.7 Non-Transport and Transport Service Name or ID Number—Name and ID number of each prehospital service assessing and/or transporting the trauma victim.

.4.8.7.1	Faith Flight I	48C
.4.8.7.2	Florida Medical Airvac	48D
.4.8.7.3	Greater Orlando Aviation Authority	48E
.4.8.7.4	Orange County Fire Rescue	48G
.4.8.7.5	Orange County Sheriff's Aviation	48H
.4.8.7.6	Orlando Fire Department	48I
.4.8.7.7	Orlando Regional Medical Center	48J
.4.8.7.8	West Orange Memorial Hospital	48M
.4.8.7.9	American Medical Transport	48O

229.0 General Information about the Trauma Scorecard
.1 Trauma Scorecard—This provides a criterion that will establish a standard for assessing the condition of the patient by using the Glasgow Trauma Score.
.1.1 All trauma patients will receive a Glasgow Trauma Score.
.1.2 Transport to a trauma center by the following criteria:
.1.2.1 Respiratory rate of 10/min or less or greater than 29/min.
.1.2.2 Systolic blood pressure of less than 90 mmHg.
.1.2.3 Glasgow Coma Score of less than 13.
.1.3 Assess the mechanism of injury:
.1.3.1 Any penetrating injuries proximal to the elbow or knee;
.1.3.2 Second- or third-degree burns involving 15% or greater BSA;
.1.3.3 Facial or airway burns;
.1.3.4 Two or more proximal long bone fractures;
.1.3.5 Limb paralysis;
.1.3.6 Amputation proximal to the wrist or ankle;

.1.3.7 Ejection from an automobile;
.1.3.8 Death of another occupant in the same automobile;
.1.3.9 Extrication time of greater than 20 minutes;

1. PATIENT'S NAME	2. SEX	3. DOB or AGE	4. RACE	5. WT./KG	6. RES.	PRIVATE PHYSICIAN

7. PATIENT'S ADDRESS	8. RUN NUMBER	9.	10. AGY	11. STN	UNIT	DEST. DET.

12. INCIDENT LOCATION	13. RUN DATE	14. S.T.R	15. DUP	POLICE

16. CALL REC'D	23. MILEAGE	24. TYPE OF CALL	33. NATURE OF RUN
17. UNIT ENRT	TO	25. DISP. OF CALL	
18. ARR'VD LOC	FROM	26. PT TAKEN TO	34. PROTOCOL USED
19. ARR'VD PT	TOTAL	27. EXTRICATION	
20. PT DEP'D	39. ALS	28. SEAT BELT	ALLERGIES
21. ARR'VD DEST	40. ARRHYTHMIA	29. CHILD RESTR.	
22. UNIT AVAIL.		30. HELMET	
		31. ANATOMY OF INJ.	
35. ATTENDANT A		32. GLASGOW COMA SCORE	REPORT RECEIVED
36. ATTENDANT B			PHYSICIAN'S SIGNATURE
37. OTHER O			
38. OTHER O			

BEAR DOWN WHILE WRITING
ALL COPIES MUST BE LEGIBLE

COMMENTS:

TIME	L.O.C.	B.P.	P	R	CC/EKG	TREATMENT	RESPONSE	AID/ATT

SIGNATURE: DATE:

40-1 (8/88) ORANGE COUNTY, FLORIDA, EMS

6 RES.
Y-YES
N-NO

15 DUP.
Y-YES
N-NO

24 TYPE OF CALL
A EMERGENCY
B NON EMERGENCY
C PUBLIC SERVICE

25 DISP. OF CALL
A TRANSP
B TRANSF
C TREAT O
D EXAM O
E STANDBY
F FALSE CALL
G DRY RUN
H CX

26 PT TAKEN TO
A FLA ORL
B FLA ALT
C FLA APK
D B.C.H.
E O.R.M.C.
F SANDLAKE
G ORL GEN
H WEST ORG
I WINTER PARK
J HUMANA LUC
K NAVAL HOSP
L RESIDENCE
M NURSING HOME
N OTHER

27 EXTRICATION
TIME

28 SEAT BELT
Y-YES
N-NO

29 CHILD RESTRAINT
Y-YES
N-NO

30 HELMET
Y-YES
N-NO

31 ANATOMY OF INJURY
A. 2°/3° BURNS > 15% BSA
B. PARALYSIS
C. AMPUTATION PROX. TO WRIST OR ANKLE
D. EJECTION FROM AUTO
E. PENETRATING INJURY TO HEAD, NECK, CHEST, ABDOMEN, OR GROIN

32 GLASGOW COMA SCALE

MOTOR RESPONSE	
OBEYS COMMAND	6
LOCALIZES PAIN	5
WITHDRAW (PAIN)	4
FLEXION (PAIN)	3
EXTENSION (PAIN)	2
NONE	1
EYE OPENING	
SPONTANEOUS	4
TO VOICE	3
TO PAIN	2
NONE	1
VERBAL RESPONSE	
ORIENTED	5
CONFUSED	4
INAPPROPRIATE WORDS	3
INCOMPREHENSIBLE WORDS	2
NONE	1
DESIGNATION	
<13 LEVEL I TRAUMA CENTER	

DESTINATION DETERMINED BY:
A PT REQUEST
B FAMILY REQUEST
C PHYSICIAN REQUEST
D NEAREST APPROPRIATE FACILITY FOR PT'S COND.

33 NATURE OF RUN
A AUTO
B MOTORCYCLE
C BICYCLE
D PED.
E ASSAULT
F NEAR-DROWNING
G FALL
H FIRE/BURN
I AIRCRAFT
J OB
K G.S.W.
L STAB.
M LAC/ABRAS
N AMPUT
O FRACT
P ELECT
Q CARDIAC
R ETOH
S SEIZ.
T DYSPNEA
U C.V.A.
V OD/POIS.
W PSYCH
X SUICIDE
Y DIABETIC
Z EXPIRED
XX PATIENT SAVE
ZZ GENERAL ILLNESS
YY MINOR TRAUMA
WW UNRESPONSIVE

34 PROTOCOL USED
A STANDING ORDERS
B PHYSICIANS ORDERS
C GEN/MED
D GEN/TR
E A.M.I.
F P.E.
G ARREST
H DYSRHYTHMIA
I BP
J C.V.A.
K DIABETIC
L OBST. AIRWAY
M ASTHMA
N UNCONSCIOUS
O TOX/EXP/OVER DOSE
P SEIZ
Q PSYCH
R SHOCK
S MULTI TR.
T HEAD TR.
U SPINAL TR.
V EYE TR.
W CHEST TR.
X ABD TR.
Y EXT TR.
Z BURNS
A2 RAPE
B2 TEMP
C2 BIRTH
D2 PEDS
E2 DEATH

35 AID TO THE PT
A IV-EXTREMITY
B IV-EXT JUG
C DRUG THERAPY
D OXYGEN
E ETT-ORAL
F ETT-NASAL
G EOA
H CRIC. STAB
I M.A.S.T.
J DEFIB/CARD
K EXT PACER
L CPR
M CITIZEN CPR
N SPINE/NECK IMMOB.
O TX/SPLINT
P BAND/CONT BLEED
Q NITROUS OXIDE
R CARD MONITOR
S EXAM
T OB/DELIV.
U PLEURAL DECOMP
V COLD APPLICATION
W SUCTIONING
X B-V-M/VENT
Y FLUID CHALLENGE

38 ALS
Y-YES
N-NO

40 ARRHYTHMIA
1. NSR
2. SINUS TACH
3. BRADY
4. A-FIB
5. A FLUT
6. ASYSTOLE
7. VF
8. VT
9. 1°
10. MOB I
11. MOB II
12. 3°
13. AGONAL
14. OTHER
15. P.V.C.'s
16. E.M.D.

Pediatric Drug dosages
a. Sodium Bicarbonate 1meg/kg.
(1). Up to 5kg use 4.2% or .5meq/ml.
(2). 6 – 50kg. use 8.4% or 1meq/ml.
b. Epinephrine .01mg/kg.
c. Atropine .02 – .03mg/kg. (max – .5/dose)
d. Lidocaine 0.5 – 1mg/kg
e. CaCl 10% – 10mg/kg (.1cc)
f. Valium 0.3 – 0.5mg/kg (max. – 10mg.)
g. Dextrose 25% – 4cc/kg.
h. Narcan – 0.01mg/kg.
i. Lasix – 1mg/kg.
j. Bretylium – 5mg/kg.
k. Ipecac – 6-12 months – 10cc
1-5 years – 15cc
over 5 years – 30cc

Pediatric IV Drips
a. Dopamine (40mg/cc)
Add 3.75cc to 250cc D5W
1cc/kg/hr. = 10mcq/kg/min.
(dose – 5-10mcq/kg/min)
b. Lidocaine (20mg/cc)
Add 15cc to 250cc D5W
1cc/kg/hr = 20mcq/kg/min.
(dose – 20-50mcq/kg/min.)

RULES OF NINE

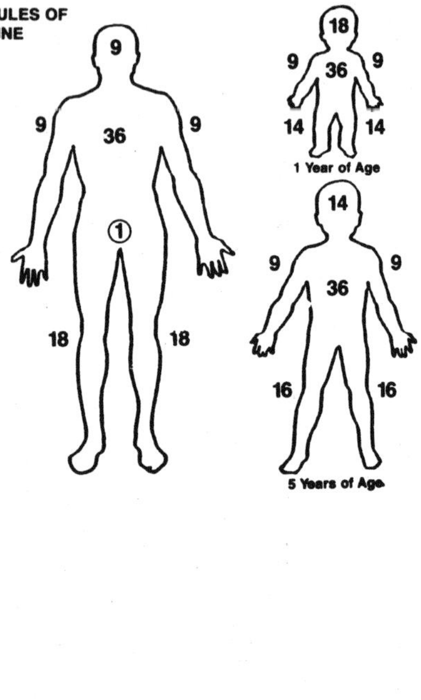

APGAR SCORE

Category	VALUE 0	VALUE 1	VALUE 2
Heart rate	absent	<100	>100
Respirations	absent	slow irregular	good w/cry
Muscle tone	flaccid	poor	good. with spontaneous movement
Reflexes, Irritability	No reflex motion	grimace	cry
Color	Cyanotic	body pink. extremities cyanotic	pink